WAR AND THE MILITARIZATION OF BRITISH ARMY MEDICINE, 1793–1830

STUDIES FOR THE SOCIETY FOR THE SOCIAL HISTORY
OF MEDICINE

Series Editors: *David Cantor*
                   Keir Waddington

TITLES IN THIS SERIES

1 Meat, Medicine and Human Health in the Twentieth Century
David Cantor, Christian Bonah and Matthias Dörries (eds)

2 Locating Health: Historical and Anthropological Investigations
of Place and Health
Erika Dyck and Christopher Fletcher (eds)

3 Medicine in the Remote and Rural North, 1800–2000
J. T. H. Connor and Stephan Curtis (eds)

4 A Modern History of the Stomach: Gastric Illness, Medicine and British
Society, 1800–1950
Ian Miller

WAR AND THE MILITARIZATION OF BRITISH ARMY MEDICINE, 1793–1830

BY

Catherine Kelly

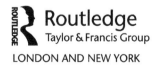

Routledge
Taylor & Francis Group

LONDON AND NEW YORK

First published 2011 by Pickering & Chatto (Publishers) Limited

Published 2016 by Routledge
2 Park Square, Milton Park, Abingdon, Oxfordshire OX14 4RN
711 Third Avenue, New York, NY 10017, USA

First issued in paperback 2015

Routledge is an imprint of the Taylor & Francis Group, an informa business

BRITISH LIBRARY CATALOGUING IN PUBLICATION DATA

Kelly, Catherine, 1974–
War and the militarization of British Army medicine, 1793–1830. – (Studies for the Society for the Social History of Medicine)
1. Medicine, Military – Great Britain – History – 18th century. 2. Medicine, Military – Great Britain – History – 19th century. 3. Great Britain. Army – Medical personnel – History – 18th century. 4. Great Britain. Army – Medical personnel – History – 19th century. 5. Physicians – Great Britain – History – 19th century. 6. Medicine – Great Britain – History – 19th century. 7. Napoleonic Wars, 1800–1815 – Medical care. 8. Medicine, Military – France – History –18th century.
I. Title II. Series
616.9'8023'0941'09033-dc22

ISBN-13: 978-1-138-66159-2 (pbk)
ISBN-13: 978-1-8489-3183-1 (hbk)
Typeset by Pickering & Chatto (Publishers) Limited

CONTENTS

ACKNOWLEDGEMENTS

This project would never have been completed without the very generous support of the Wellcome Trust, and the support, inspiration and guidance I found at the Wellcome Unit for the History of Medicine in Oxford. First and foremost thanks must go to Mark Harrison who sparked my interest in the medicine of this period with an evocative description of the activities of Charles Maclean. Throughout my doctoral studies, and in the revision and extension of the manuscript for publication, he was an endless source of advice, reassurance, and inspiration. Margaret Pelling has been enormously generous with her time and advice and always made me think harder. I am particularly grateful to Joanna Innes, and Laurence Brockliss who shared with me their insights into the medicine, army, and politics of the Napoleonic Wars. This volume has benefited greatly from the comments and suggestions of Harold Cooke, Lisa Rosner, Geoffrey Hudson and Keir Waddington. My thanks also to Carol Brady and Belinda Michaelides who went out of their way on countless occasions to assist me.

In the course of my research I have incurred many debts to numerous colleagues and friends. I was extremely fortunate to have been provided with a home in London by Shankari Chandran whose support in all endeavours over the past twenty years has been invaluable. Similarly, numerous research trips were made possible by Jessica Sansom, Lyndon Coppin, Nerilee Telford, Davinia Caddy, Chris Bradley, Isabel Back, and Lynette Basha, who all welcomed me into their homes on many occasions. I am also very grateful to Erica Charters, Merridee Bailey, Gaurav Gaiha, Imogen Goold, Ryan Johnson and Rod Nicholls for their comments, suggestions, support and friendship. For help with my French, thanks must go to Gemma Betros. I am also indebted to the often anonymous staff and archivists of The Wellcome Library, The British Library, The Bodleian Library, The National Archives, The University of Glasgow, and the Apothecaries Hall for the efficient, helpful, and vital service they have provided.

To my grandparents Tom and Joan Kelly, Rita King, and my great-aunt Florence Jackson, my sister Jane and brother Tim, and especially to my parents, Barbara and John, I will be eternally grateful for the love, opportunities, and encouragement they have given me all my life. More recently, I have been lucky to have the love and partnership of my husband, Jason, who I met close to the beginning of this project and who has supported me in many important ways throughout. And to my daughter Tabitha, who I met near the end, for everything she has brought into my life.

ABBREVIATIONS

The following abbreviations have been used throughout the volume:

AMB   Army Medical Board
AMD   Army Medical Department
Wars   The French Revolutionary and Napoleonic Wars

NOTE ON THE TEXT

Original spelling and punctuation have been retained in quotations; '*sic*' has been used only where the original quotation could suggest an error of accuracy.

The terms 'inquiry' and 'enquiry' were used interchangeably during the period under consideration. With the exception of the body given the official title 'The Commissioners of Military Enquiry', in all cases 'inquiry' has been used.

INTRODUCTION

During the French Revolutionary and Napoleonic Wars, British doctors travelled in unprecedented numbers to foreign and often exotic locations where they were confronted with battlefield injuries, virulent and mysterious diseases and complex military politics that few had encountered before. These experiences changed the way they viewed their profession, the nature of disease and the types of treatment that were effective. This book makes a departure from histories which depict their work as bloody, violent and futile, to examine instead how nearly twenty five years of sustained warfare affected the professional identity embraced by those doctors and thoroughly militarized their approach to medicine. I argue that the philosophy they came to embrace – that military medicine was a specialized field – was not only important to the practice of medicine within the British army, but also had significant implications for the development of medicine in nineteenth-century Britain.

Throughout the following chapters a handful of senior medical officers feature prominently as their influence on the development of military medicine is traced through their participation in campaign after campaign from 1793 to 1815. These men headed a department which expanded tenfold over the course of the Wars, providing vital opportunities for experiment and implementation of new ideas. It housed a large pool of medical recruits eager to learn and get ahead. In 1789, 152 medical officers were serving with the department; by 1814 this number had risen to 1,274. Over the entire period, 2,834 medical officers were recruited.[1] By 1800, it was not uncommon for aspiring doctors to begin their medical education with the goal of securing employment in the military. The engagement of such a significant proportion of not just one but two generations of British medical practitioners in these Wars produced a large professional group who considered that they practised a previously unarticulated specialty in military medicine, and who viewed themselves as military medical officers, distinct from, and in many ways superior to, their civilian colleagues.

The general features of this new professional identity were: a belief in the superiority of 'on-the-field training' over academic study (although not to its exclusion); a preference for empirical approaches to medicine; a challenge to the division between surgery and physic; an incorporation of the practical needs of military operations into schemes for the preservation of health; and the adoption of the military norms and values that prevailed at the time. This identity was expounded in print by leading military medical officers and came to be expressed by military practitioners in opposition to the professional claims of their civilian colleagues. It was also asserted against practitioners within the army perceived as being too civilian in their approach.

With its emphasis on an observationally-based, empirical approach, military medicine shares many of the characteristics of 'hospital medicine', identified by Erwin Ackerknecht and Michel Foucault as one of the most significant developments in the practice of modern medicine.[2] The participation of the French military in this process has received attention from historians, but the British contribution remains unexamined.[3] Equally, the genesis of military medicine in foreign climates far away from traditional centres of authority bears similarity to factors that have been shown to have influenced the development of 'tropical medicine' among practitioners who served in the East India Company and in the far reaches of Empire.[4] Both embrace a strong shift away from humoral explanations of disease instead emphasizing the role of climate in the production of illness. However, the incorporation of military values and practicalities significantly militarized both the theory and application of military medicine, giving it a cultural aspect not found in tropical or hospital medicine.

Military medicine was a medicine that was validated not just by the theories of its practitioners, but also by the army structure in which it developed, and by the patients on whom it was practised. Importantly, military medical practitioners tried to use this medicine not just to heal the sick and injured but also to advance their claims to officer status.

This book examines the emergence of this new group who identified themselves as military medical officers and considers how they influenced the way in which medicine was practised within the British army. The contribution of military medicine to wider changes in medicine during the nineteenth century, and the impact of military practitioners on the British medical profession, is assessed in the final part of the book which examines the efforts of military and ex-military practitioners to promote their approach and expertise after the Wars to both their civilian colleagues and potential patients.

There is a large body of scholarship that identifies the eighteenth and early nineteenth centuries as an era in which British medicine experienced significant upheaval.[5] However, there has been no comprehensive investigation of the contribution made to these changes by medical officers serving with the British army. John Pickstone stated that to understand fully what happened to British medicine during this period, several 'key medical milieux' needed comprehensive investigation. In particular, he believed that 'we have hardly begun to work out the consequences' of Britain's participation in the French Revolutionary and Napoleonic Wars.[6] In a more recent work, Geoffrey Hudson puts forward an argument that British military medicine of this period remains seriously under-researched.[7]

The changes in British medicine during this period are usually associated with the development of hospitals, the rise of the general practitioner, pathological anatomy and the emergence of clinical trials and medical statistics. Although the contribution of British military practitioners has not received the attention it deserves, it has been noted that military hospitals were at the forefront of developments in other processes that strongly valued observation and lesion-based theories of disease, such as morbid anatomy, and the mass observation of patients.[8] Additionally, much of the impetus behind new forms of knowledge during this period is thought to have come from the extremities of the Empire. William Bynum has argued that overseas medical practitioners had an instrumental role in promoting the discussion and adoption of new ideas, particularly in relation to fever.[9] Historians who have considered the British military dimension to developments in medicine have generally concentrated on the seventeenth and early eighteenth centuries. They have demonstrated that the exigencies of war and the desire of practitioners to enhance their status within the services may have influenced the type of medicine they pursued. Harold Cook has shown that, following the reorganization of the Army Medical Service by William III and Mary II in the late seventeenth century, the military leadership demanded specific medicines that would be widely efficacious for specific diseases. This demand was contrary to received medical theory at the time, which asserted that 'no disease was precisely the same in every patient'.[10] The effect of the British military establishment's growing interest in 'curative medicine further legitimized the increasingly respectable medical empiricism'.[11] In addition, Cook argues, harried practitioners on military service would have embraced such an approach to medicine as it was practicable in the circumstances they faced, and more desirable to their immediate military commanders.

Similarly, an increasing interest in preventative medicine, or hygienic medicine, among naval practitioners has been identified by Christopher Lawrence during the period 1750–1825, when the management of disease was vital to imperial expansion. Lawrence makes the twofold argument that the advocacy by naval practitioners of disciplinary measures to encourage good health, such as the divisional system implemented in the 1790s, was motivated both by a desire to increase their importance (and thus status) within the service, as well as reflecting emerging ideas about social organization.[12] In the following chapters it will be shown how similar factors were influential in the development of medical theory among army medical officers during and after the Wars, thus demonstrating not only the changes that took place within British military medicine but also the continuities that persisted.

Naval medicine during the Wars has been written about extensively. The organization of the AMD, the conditions in which military medical officers worked and the multiple interactions they had with military officers produced a culture, and administrative and medical challenges significantly different to those that prevailed in the Navy. While there are certainly many analogies between the two services, and collaborations between military and naval medical officers were relatively common, the particular environment in which army medical officers worked was integral to the production of the military medical officer identity and concept of military medicine. This is the principal focus of this study. While contemporary comparisons between the two services, and collaborations between them, are considered in the following chapters, this book only touches lightly on Naval medicine during the Wars.[13]

The work of the AMD during this period has been well chronicled by historians such as Neil Cantlie, Richard Blanco, and Martin Howard who have written thorough treatments of the administrative arrangements of the service, also addressing the quality of medical recruits, deployment of troops and medical officers, the medical and surgical treatments used and the military rank or status of medical practitioners.[14] They generally agree that the Wars allowed or forced the army medical service to become significantly more expert and effective than it had been prior to 1793. In particular, they argue that improvements were achieved in the technical (mostly surgical) skills of the medical practitioners, and in the logistic and administrative skills of the men heading the department and its divisions. However, these medical histories to a lesser or greater extent fail to consider contemporary medicine on its own terms or evaluate it in that context. The conclusion that army doctors made no major discoveries in the classification or treatment of disease, were confused by ancient theories of disease causation, and that effective treatments were fortuitous, is common to these histories.[15] Those same conclusions are repeated in military histories of the Wars, which are usually limited to giving lurid accounts of battlefield surgery and setting out the losses from disease suffered by the army.[16]

More recently, historians have exploded traditional military medical histories that dismissed these practitioners as ill-educated butchers purveying a medicine based on misguided science. The successes of disease prevention during this period were based on more than a fortuitous alignment of circumstance. Additionally, historians have begun to illuminate the ways in which new forms of medical evidence and reporting were constructed by these practitioners.[17] It has also been shown that they did all these things within a context in which it was necessary to cultivate military or political patronage to succeed. Crucially, recent scholarship has established a profile of the typical recruit to the medical service and proved that his education was not, as held in popular mythology, woefully inadequate.[18] It has been established that the army medical service was a window of social opportunity for those from relatively humble backgrounds, particularly those from the Celtic fringe. The average recruit was most likely to be Scottish, or from a rural area, and to have come from one of a wide variety of middling backgrounds most likely in trade or agriculture. He was most often a 'lower order' son. While he was well educated, probably having passed through a grammar school, apprenticeship and at least one or two years of university medical courses, he was still 'relatively disadvantaged compared with other entrants to the medical marketplace'[19] and for that reason probably chose to enter the military service.

However, the question of whether recruits to the AMD were as well educated as some of their peers was still a burning issue in the early nineteenth century. A major argument of this book is that the framing of military medicine as a skilled specialization arose partly in response to aspersions cast upon the education of medical officers who had begun their careers in the army and roadblocks placed in the path of their career advancement because of such claims. Significantly, this claim was made half a century prior to the usual chronology attributed to the rise of medical specialization.[20]

The type of medical education these recruits would have received has been investigated in studies by Irvine Loudon and Susan Lawrence. They demonstrate the increasing dominance of teaching hospitals and university departments of medicine. During this period ever increasing numbers of young practitioners came to believe there was value in attending large hospitals, particularly in London, and walking the wards as a part of their medical education. Gradually the hospital became the site for teaching and research, and this process ultimately vested medical authority in hospital men and 'men of science', and in argumentative forms favouring the 'objective' based on an 'undisguised commitment to a descriptive empiricism'.[21] Students who went on to serve as medical officers in the AMD were active participants in the new forms of medical education, attending lectures at Edinburgh and in London, also taking up opportunities to walk the wards in teaching hospitals.[22] It is probable that this background pre-disposed those men to readily accept the value of bedside observation and to turn to an empirical, experimental, medicine when faced with the challenges of practice on campaign.

However, these two branches of historical inquiry have not been brought together. Lawrence and Loudon give cursory attention to students destined for the military, but in broader studies of the changes to British medicine during this period, the reader could be forgiven for not realizing that Britain was at war. If we are to fully understand the changes which occurred in British medicine during this period the experience and influence of practitioners who served with the military must be properly investigated. A primary aim of this book is to establish the effects of service in the AMD during the Wars on the professional development and medical theories of military medical officers. In addition those findings will be placed within the broader context of changes to British medicine during the first half of the nineteenth century.

This book is not a comprehensive examination of every aspect of the army medical service, or of the Wars themselves. The campaigns that have been selected for examination are some of the most strategically significant in which Britain participated; those with little relevance to the development of the military medical officer have been omitted. The most glaring omission is the campaign known as the 100 Days, culminating at the Battle of Waterloo. Despite the importance of the battle to the ultimate victory of Britain in the Wars, the medical arrangements for the campaign were hastily made, notoriously ineffective, and while important to the development of some surgical techniques, close examination of them adds little new material to the conclusions about military medical officers reached in the chapters on earlier campaigns.

Chapter 1 addresses the early campaigns of the Wars in the Low Countries and the West Indies. In both those theatres, the British army was ravaged by fever. The campaigns were formative for several of the practitioners who appear as key players throughout the following chapters, including James McGrigor, William Fergusson and Robert Jackson. The chapter demonstrates how disputes over promotion within the service, challenges to the authority of the AMB, and wrangling over the control of the medical arrangements for various expeditions, caused practitioners to reconsider their claims for status within the army. The new medical challenges and unfamiliar diseases they faced also caused these practitioners to question what they had previously learned, and contributed to the development of claims that 'military diseases' and 'military medicine' were distinct from those encountered in civilian practice. It will also be shown how the relationship between military and medical needs was perceived by military leaders, and why medical practitioners wedded to older forms of knowledge and practice were gradually to lose the battle to define the course of British military medicine as the Wars progressed. The chapter concludes that by the end of these campaigns two important trends had begun to emerge in British army medicine: an attempt to articulate a distinct military medical specialty; and a struggle by medical practitioners to adapt to a military framework, often alongside attempts to manipulate it to obtain medical power.

Debates over the existence of a 'military medical specialty' are further considered in Chapter 2. This chapter examines conflicts between old-school practitioners and the emerging 'military medical officers', which culminated in a parliamentary inquiry into the Walcheren expedition in 1809. The inquiry has been seen as the catalyst for the demise of the AMB. That conclusion is questioned, and it is demonstrated that the demise of the Board was in fact the result of a long-standing deterioration of its relationship with its own medical practitioners, and with the military command. By examining the disintegration of the AMB over the period from its inception to 1810, it will be shown that debates about military medicine were not driven solely by an intellectual commitment to particular theories of disease. While arguing about appropriate medical practice, medical practitioners were also striving to assert and control competing visions of the future of the medical profession; a future in which they perceived there would be a limited market for medical services. At their heart, almost all the medical debates entered into during this period within the AMD were about the competing claims of the two models of medical education, and the consequent issue of whether army medical practice required specialized training. Ironically, the ultimate effect of these debates was the erosion of military medicine's professional autonomy as Parliament was forced to step in and, in effect, decide medical debates.

Chapter 3 considers more deeply how medical practice in a foreign climate contributed to the production of the notion that military medicine was specialized and distinct from civilian practice. This chapter investigates that process through a detailed examination of the Egyptian campaign that began with the French invasion of Egypt in 1798. On that campaign, both armies were afflicted with severe and persistent dysentery and medical practitioners were confronted by a harsh and unfamiliar climate that appeared to produce diseases of which they had almost no experience, such as the plague and Egyptian ophthalmia. The writings of practitioners on the campaign are used to demonstrate how army doctors approached the 'new' diseases, giving some insight into the investigative processes and medical philosophies of these men. In particular, new ways in which Dr James McGrigor was able to use the military system to control, direct and disseminate the development of medical knowledge is considered. It is concluded that these intellectual processes and philosophies were important building blocks in the construction of army medical officers' argued positions in later debates over their medical superiority to civilian practitioners.

The spread of Egyptian ophthalmia throughout the British army when it returned to Britain is examined in the second half of this chapter. It shows how a growing identification of the disease with filth and contagion superseded climatic theories of disease that had previously been favoured, and how debates over appropriate treatment began to highlight potential conflict between military and civilian practitioners. Finally, the chapter investigates the attempts of senior army medical officers to control and standardize the treatment of the disease.

Chapters 4 and 5 consider the Peninsular War and demonstrate how and why army medicine and army medical officers became increasingly militarized. In particular, the implications for the development of army medicine resulting from the appointment of the new AMB are discussed. By examining the relative success and failure of the most senior military medical officers on the Peninsular service, these chapters highlight how important it had become for medical officers to adapt their practice to accommodate not only the practicalities of campaigning, but also the values of army culture.

Chapter 4 focuses on the tragic Corunna campaign and the first half of the Peninsular War. It shows how the increasing demand for qualified hospital mates affected the professional aspirations of young medical students, and how it reinforced the concept that 'on-the-field' training was at least as relevant to an army medical career as a traditional medical education. The varying approaches of the senior medical officers on these campaigns are examined, and through them the widespread adoption of military norms within army medical practice is adduced, as is an emerging consolidation of medical philosophy among the officers of the AMD. The particular example of British medical practitioners in the Portuguese medical service shows how military practitioners continued to define themselves in opposition to (perceived) civilian prejudices against their expertise.

Chapter 5 considers the second half of the Peninsular War, with particular reference to the importance of McGrigor's role at the head of medical staff. It reconsiders the traditional account of McGrigor's time in the Peninsula – particularly his relationship with Wellington. The ways in which McGrigor tried to recruit Wellington to his cause are investigated, as is their consequent effect on the further militarization of army medicine and promotion of the 'military medical officer identity'.

The final chapter examines the impact of the Wars on the practice of medicine in Britain in the first half of the nineteenth century. In particular, the previously un-researched efforts of McGrigor to use army medical officers stationed around the globe to conduct experiments and develop consensus about appropriate therapeutics are investigated. His efforts had significant effects on both the treatment of certain diseases and the status of military medicine within British medicine more generally.

McGrigor's appointment to the head of the AMD meant that he was placed at the centre of a global network of military medical officers. He expanded the role as the hub of a knowledge network he had adopted throughout his medical career. It allowed him to attempt to adopt a role in the field of medicine similar to that which had been held by Sir Joseph Banks in the natural sciences. Chapter 6 undertakes a review of his correspondence in the first few years after the Wars and demonstrates that his efforts to promote the medical discoveries of the Wars and of practitioners serving in distant climates were strenuous. He was cognizant of the benefit that would accrue to the service if the heroic efforts of his officers were made known to the public. In this regard he encouraged the publication of several tracts about the Battle of Waterloo by military medical officers. In addition to the well-known efforts McGrigor made to encourage medical officers to pursue opportunities for further medical education following the peace, he also set about disseminating the accumulated medical experience and findings the medical department had gathered during the Wars. McGrigor was eager to forward the enquiries of prominent medical practitioners about certain diseases to the medical men who remained in the Peninsula, and on station elsewhere around the globe. He also made the documents of the medical department open to any 'professional gentleman' who might wish to consult them. One of the most important medical discoveries to come out of the Peninsular War was the Portuguese treatment of syphilis without mercury. McGrigor strongly encouraged investigation of the treatment and supported the trials being made in various quarters.

After the Wars, efforts to promote the authority of 'military medicine' led to the involvement of the British Parliament with military medicine. This chapter makes a particular investigation of the tool most often used to do this—parliamentary select committees of inquiry. A significant number of these were held into medical debates during and after the Wars and they had important implications for military medicine. The first part of the chapter demonstrates how the concept of military medicine as a distinct form of practice was brought to the attention of Parliament early in the Wars, and how parliamentarians became exposed to characteristic forms of military medical rhetoric. The latter part of the chapter examines two 'flash points' between civilian and military medical officers, and the competition for employment between them following the Wars. This is done by investigating a parliamentary inquiry into Egyptian ophthalmia and two inquiries into the plague in the 1820s. The disputes aired during those inquiries demonstrate how and why military medical practitioners asserted their identity and superiority to their civilian counterparts. The intervention of non-medical power players in the development of British medicine is also explored.

In an important departure from the historiography of British military medicine, this book seeks to understand what effects the Wars had on the medical and professional philosophies of army medical officers. It does so by considering the accounts of their service: their official and personal letters, diaries, published writings, and the arguments they used during official investigations. In so doing, the myriad and often vitriolic disputes within the medical service, between medical and civilian practitioners, between medical practitioners and army officers, and those in which politicians became involved, are uncovered. In analysing those disputes the medical practitioners' modes of rhetoric, motivations, and strategies for recruiting allies are closely examined.

The book concludes that British military practitioners must be considered active participants in the seismic shifts in medical theory during the nineteenth century. By the end of the Wars, a large group of practitioners had emerged who considered themselves to be 'military medical officers'. As a professional body they had militarized themselves, and their medicine, and considered themselves a distinct professional body from their civilian counterparts. Throughout the Wars they had engaged in debates with civilian practitioners about many issues which all, ultimately, revolved around the central question of what type of knowledge should be considered most probative in medical debates. They deliberately attacked and sought to undermine the existing sites of medical authority. The empirical and observational model advocated by military medical officers underpinned their claims to authority and expertise and, after the Wars, for marketplace space over civilian practitioners. They pursued these claims not only intra-professionally, but also in appeals to the 'public' and in the parliamentary forum. By doing so they brought their debates outside the medical sphere and ceded some authority in the development of British medicine to non-medical experts who are likely to have been more receptive to evidence based on empirical and observational models. Through all these means, the medical practitioners who served in the British army during the Wars had a significant impact on the development of British medicine.

1 THE LOW COUNTRIES AND THE WEST INDIES

Sir John Fortescue described the work of the British army in the first ten years of the Wars as 'vast ... thankless ... and unprofitable'.[1] His assessment might well have been shared by many of the medical officers who laboured during those years in difficult and disease-ridden environments, overseeing the deaths of large numbers of soldiers, for little apparent strategic gain. The West Indian expeditions of the years 1793–8 have, in particular, attracted the attention of historians for their appalling death rates among British troops.[2] These expeditions have also been identified by historians of medicine as an important contributor to the development of a distinct empirical and experimental approach to medicine particular to the tropics,[3] and to the reform of the AMD.[4] In contrast, the other major British military undertaking of the period, the Duke of York's campaigns in the Low Countries during the years 1793–5, has been largely ignored by historians both military and medical.[5] However, the campaigns in the Low Countries were fundamental to the ways in which British military medicine, and the self-image of British army medical officers, developed over the course of the Wars.

The campaigns in the Low Countries began in February 1793 when France declared war on Britain and Holland. Britain responded by entering an alliance with Austria and Prussia to protect the neutrality of Holland and to maintain the free access of shipping in the Scheldt. A meagre force of 2,500 British men was embarked under the leadership of Frederick Augustus, Duke of York. Those men joined a force of 100,000 Dutch and Austrian soldiers and British-funded Hessian and Hanoverian mercenaries. The allied army achieved some success against the French in 1793, but in 1794 (despite an influx of recruits) both the British and Austrian forces suffered a series of defeats. Towards the end of the year, the British forces carried out their retreat, ill provisioned and practically naked, in appalling winter conditions with dramatically rising numbers of sick troops. This desperate state of affairs continued throughout the first few months of 1795, until on 8 March the British Cabinet decided to withdraw from the Continent.

What little historical attention the campaigns of 1793–5 have received has not been very positive. Cantlie concluded that 'the campaign ended in disaster to the British Army, and a disaster for the Medical Department'.[6] Fortescue made serious criticisms of many aspects of the campaign but left his most damning for the medical arrangements, stating that, 'the very worst department of them all was that of the hospitals, wherein the abuses were so terrible that men hardly liked to speak of them'; and that the department comprised a 'medical staff ... improvised out of drunken apothecaries, broken down practitioners, and rogues of every description, who were provided under some cheap contract'.[7]

Fortescue's condemnation appears to have been based on opinions expressed by several military officers in letters written during the campaign. As will be seen, his conclusion is not supported by the evidence. However, it remains that contemporaries perceived the medical services provided during this campaign to have been woefully inadequate. Sickness rates were high, particularly in the latter stages of the campaign when troops suffered principally from a contagious fever.[8] As mortality rates in the general hospitals appeared to rise inexorably, tensions within the medical department grew.[9] The resulting infighting of the medical staff was considered unforgivable by military officers who blamed it for the rising death rate. However, as Cantlie noted, many of the medical department's failings were actually the fault of poor logistical planning by military leaders and unworkable policies enforced by the AMB. Many medical men who were to become influential later in the Wars, including James McGrigor, William Fergusson and Robert Jackson, served on these campaigns, and the lessons they took from the chaos on the Continent were to have a profound impact on the development of military medicine.

This chapter will consider the numerous conflicts over the control of the medical arrangements of the army that were entered into during the Low Countries campaigns. It will demonstrate that by the end of these campaigns two important trends had begun to emerge in British army medicine: an attempt to articulate a distinct military medical specialty; and a struggle by medical practitioners to adapt to a military framework, alongside attempts to manipulate it to obtain medical power. The chapter will go on to examine how those trends, which became dominant features of the army medical culture for the rest of the Wars, were reinforced by innovations in medical theory and were enhanced when the medical practitioners who had served in the Low Countries encountered the particular disease environment of the West Indies.

Military versus Civilian Practitioners

At the commencement of hostilities, the AMD was headed by the physician general, Sir Clifton Winteringham and the surgeon general, John Hunter.[10] Owing to Winteringham's advanced age and incapacity, in practice Hunter ran the AMD. Following Hunter's death in October 1793 a new AMB was appointed, comprising Surgeon General Mr John Gunning; Inspector General Thomas Keate; and (following the death of Winteringham in January 1794) Physician General Sir Lucas Pepys.[11]

The failings of the medical department in the Low Countries can be attributed to a multitude of factors, including the constantly changing military command of the general hospitals and the logistical difficulties of providing medical care throughout a continuous retreat. But the greatest contributing factor to the failures of the medical staff was the decision of the new AMB to appoint civilian physicians (that is, physicians who had not been brought up through the AMD) to run the general hospitals.[12] This practice was particularly aggravating to military surgeons because it was the reverse of Hunter's policy which had applied when many of them had joined the army, and only came into force after the campaign was already underway.

At the start of the campaign, Hunter had written to the commander-in-chief, Lord Jeffrey Amherst, setting out his policy on the selection and promotion of medical officers which required that surgeons should serve a sort of apprenticeship in the medical service of the army and work their way up through the ranks:

> When I had the Honour of my present Appointment I wished very much there should be some system of promotion ... which was that Gentlemen of that profession should begin with Mateships of regiments, that they should be promoted to Hospital Mateships; from Hospital mate to be Regimental Surgeons; from Regimental Surgeons to the Staff, either as Surgeons, or Apothecaries, and from that Station on the Staff to be Physicians, Purveyors, &c ... I have never once allowed my Friendship for any one to make me break through that rule, nor have I allowed the Solicitation of my best Friends, much my superiors, to make me recede from it.

Very importantly, Hunter went on to state that application of that policy had positively affected recruitment into the army and established clear career expectations for the army surgeon:

> Since the above plan has been adopted, and most religiously executed on my part, the Physical Gentlemen of the Army have looked up to me as their protector, and I am certain many have entered as mates of Regiments upon the Faith of regular promotion that would not otherwise have entered and I could wish to keep their Confidence with me.[13]

Following Hunter's death, those expectations were dealt a devastating blow. Shortly after their appointment, Keate wrote to Gunning criticizing the system of promotion, suggesting that it favoured 'old Regimental Surgeons' who should more properly decorate the superannuated list.[14] The AMB members devised a new plan which they described as 'the reverse of our predecessor ... to make Physicians of Gentlemen bred to Physick, and Hospital Surgeons of Men bred to Surgery'.[15]

The new approach of the AMB set 'civilian' and 'military' medical men in the army against each other, as it considered 'Gentlemen bred to Physick' to be civilian practitioners who held a degree in medicine from a select group of universities, effectively debarring military surgeons from promotion. This caused military practitioners at all levels to consider their qualifications and assert their various claims to professional competence in ways they had not been required to do in the past.

The AMB's attitude to the regimental surgeon was hardly novel. The shortcomings of regimental surgeons had become a point of comment in medical literature, and in the correspondence of the AMB before this time.[16] The general complaint against the regimental surgeon's education was put forward by Dr Robert Hamilton in his *Duties of a Regimental Surgeon* published in 1794. He argued that although some had received a 'proper' medical education at a university 'many more have ... find [*sic*] their way into it thro' *interest* and misapplied *recommendation*',[17] and that others had been admitted who were merely 'boys who have served in the shop of some country apothecary only a year or two, nay it may be only a few months'.[18] His further objection related to the inadequacy of their training whilst serving with the army. Hamilton believed a university education was necessary to absorb and understand what the young surgeon saw on service.[19]

The new AMB was not entirely hostile to regimental surgeons. In fact, the AMB was zealous in protecting their financial interests through promotion to non-medically active positions such as apothecaryships and purveyorships as a reward for long service.[20] Many older regimental surgeons may have been content with that arrangement; however, for the young men recently entered into the medical service, and those who were to follow them, the denigration of the regimental surgeon's abilities was devastating. What was most significant, to the men of the medical service, was the clear statement that previous lines of promotion would be denied them, and those men not 'bred to physick' could not ever expect to become military physicians. This attitude was in direct contrast to the writings of leading military practitioners who had previously acknowledged the blurring of boundaries between physic and surgery in military practice. Even Hamilton had said, we all know that regimental practice partakes more of the physician's than the surgeon's province ... we oftener meet with fever, and other contagious and epidemic diseases among soldiers, than such only as need external treatment, and the hand of the operative surgeon.[21]

The policy also impeded recruitment, causing surprise to many practitioners eager to enlist as the Wars continued. The AMB records are full of letters to various doctors and surgeons informing them that without the degree of MD from a 'respectable' university or taking the examination for Licentiate of the Royal College of Physicians, they could not be appointed to the army in the position they sought.[22]

As will be seen later in this chapter, the policy was one which the AMB was constantly called on to defend to military leaders, and which it took the step of explaining in detail to the King.[23] Ultimately, the AMB defended its position by arguing that surely military commanders would want, 'Army Physicians legally authorized to practice Physic in England' – a misrepresentation of actual legal requirements to practise medicine in England.[24] The policy was also roundly criticized by several medical practitioners after the campaign. The earliest of these tracts was written in 1796 by Nathanial Sinnott who had served with the army in the Low Countries. Despite acknowledging that the circumstances were 'unfavourable ... to the forming of a perfect hospital', Sinnot argues that the accumulated miseries suffered by the unfortunate soldiers could only have come about as a result of ignorance, mismanagement or neglect. That ignorance, especially of military medical practice, he laid at the door of the hospital staff chosen by the AMB:

> Medical skill, activity and a knowledge of the oeconomy and regulation of military hospitals, constitute the chief qualifications of an army physician; and the last is more necessary, and of more consequence, than profound medical erudition. The miseries experienced by the sick did not proceed so much from a want of medical knowledge, as from a want of skill and activity in the management of our hospitals ...
>
> The Medical Board therefore, in appointing physicians to the Army, have not been sufficiently attentive to their necessary qualifications, for they have not recommended such as could possibly know any thing of military hospitals previous to their being appointed. A man directly from a university, without experience, even in physic, may be appointed physician to the army, if he become a licentiate of the College of Physicians; this is the only preparation thought necessary, and so rigidly do they adhere to this system, that if a man possessed the knowledge of Sir John Pringle, it would not recommend him so much as having a licence from the College.[25]

Dr James Borland also wrote about the impressions he had formed after the first embarkation of troops for the Continent. He had thought twice about presenting his observations to the AMB immediately following the campaign, but by 1805 had been convinced by his friends that he should do so. His stated purpose was to enquire whether 'selecting Physicians and Surgeons to the Forces from civil life is the best that can be advised for securing to His Majesty's Troops proper Medical aid in the scenes of actual war'.[26]

His reluctance to present the document earlier was most likely the consequence of his claim that the use of civilian practitioners might have been a cause of the 'dreadful mortality' experienced in the Duke of York's armies. He argued that the setting aside of regimental surgeons had had dreadful consequences, driving them out of frustrated hope to become 'idle and indolent', and that in their 'ill humour many Regimental Surgeons feeling themselves deserted were led to desert their sick and wounded'. This resulted in the soldiers being sent to military hospitals where they fell under the care of 'Medical Officers, who had never before seen a military hospital or a sick soldier'. According to Borland, civilian practitioners had been unable to enforce the appropriate military discipline in military hospitals, and the result was the generation of a contagious fever that then raged among the soldiers. He did not dispute the education of these 'college and town bred physicians' but noted that 'because they were ignorant of the peculiarities of army practice' they were ineffective on campaign. His contrasting sketch of the military practitioner was one of a resourceful man, who unlike the civilian practitioners was willing to engage in all levels of a patient's treatment. Borland also suggested that the distinction between physician and surgeon in military practice was one 'without a difference'. His argument for the distinctiveness of military medicine, was based not just on the distinct diseases suffered by soldiers, but also on the necessity in that practice of understanding the habits of soldiers, and the importance of military discipline.

The affront taken by military practitioners to the sudden elevation of civilian practitioners in the Low Countries was deeply felt, and prompted vitriolic explosions even decades after the end of the Wars:

> as physicians, setting aside their utter ignorance of diseases at so early an age, more especially military ones, they were far too fine for common use. To one of them I was attached in the first campaign ... He was my superior by at least four degrees of military rank, but I had to teach him what I myself was taught in the early days of my apprenticeship ... to have placed such men over the heads of all who were experienced in military medicine and diseases, while he was not fit for any work, was as stupid and gross an abuse as could have been imposed on any army. The assumption, the affront to every principle of service, was monstrous, and shows to what extent university and corporate pride will proceed, when unchecked by wise regulation and military rule.[27]

In these tracts we can see military practitioners attempting to articulate their particular claims to competence and the beginnings of a movement to characterize military medicine as a distinct specialty from civilian practice. In contrast to earlier works by Pringle and Monro that simply identified the diseases of soldiers on campaign as different to those of civilian life, these works singled out the experience and education of the military medical officer as also being distinct.[28] Moreover, the works of Pringle and Monro had never sought to depreciate the skill of any group of practitioners, whereas Sinnott and Borland were clearly attempting to establish an ascendancy over a group (civilian practitioners) whose education they considered inadequate. Not surprisingly, in the context of the AMB's approach to regimental surgeons, it is precisely the 'on-the-field training' such men acquired that Sinnott and Borland identified as the best preparation for an army medical career. The effects of the AMB's new policy were to become an even greater source of division later in the Wars when military surgeons refined their claims to superiority over their civilian-trained counterparts.

Other conflicts within the medical department during the campaigns in the Low Countries also had a profound effect on the development of military medical culture and the military medical officer. The need for army medical services to integrate with the priorities and requirements of the military command established conditions favouring the advancement of a new breed of medical practitioners at the higher levels. While the regimental surgeons nursed grievances against their colleagues on the ground and the AMB in London, the AMB had similar problems of its own. During the campaigns, the AMB was engaged in conflicts over control of the medical affairs of the army and struggled to convince military leaders of its superior abilities in the estimation of the skill of medical practitioners and the right to recommend them for appointments. The AMB was challenged by both old-school medical men and military leaders themselves for that right. The convoluted struggles for control of the medical arrangements of the campaigns required medical practitioners to court the favour of military leaders, something at which some practitioners were much more successful than others.

Medical Authority and Military Support

The campaign in the Low Countries was the first of its kind in almost thirty years. It presented the inexperienced AMD with logistical difficulties, obstinate military commanders, and recalcitrant physicians. Together these factors resulted in fierce disputes about authority over the medical arrangements of the army among medical men, and between medical men and military commanders. Many physicians simply could not adapt to the command structure of military life, or to the oversight of their professional activities, but nearly all began to amend their styles of argument to incorporate 'military' or 'tactical' reasoning that they hoped would appeal to their army commanders.

At the commencement of the campaigns, the then surgeon general, John Hunter, had foreseen possible conflicts between medical practitioners and had issued orders designed to prevent conflicts between physicians and surgeons in the management of the sick. His *Instructions for the Conduct of the Medical Staff Serving with the British Forces Under the Command of His R.H. the Duke of York* stated, *inter alia*, that

> Every part of management respecting the sick, whether in general or Regimental Hospital is to be govern'd by the orders of the Physicians; except that, in the treatment of cases strictly chirurgical, the surgeons are not to be subject to the countroul [*sic*] of the Physicians.[29]

Despite these instructions, infighting began soon after the arrival of the troops on the Continent and, to enforce some order, Dr Hugh Kennedy was appointed Inspector of Hospitals to the forces under the Duke of York.[30] The reasons for Kennedy's appointment are not clear from the available records. However, his disgruntlement at not being appointed to the force in the first place was definitely communicated to Lord Amherst and Hunter.[31] Once appointed, Kennedy's refusal to accept the existence of any higher medical authority than himself was to cause enormous difficulties for the AMB.

Hunter first experienced Kennedy's particular approach to his appointment soon after he arrived on the Continent. In August 1793, Hunter wrote to Lord Amherst to inform him that Kennedy had recommended two surgeons and five mates to the hospital on the Continent, and asked Amherst not to confirm one of the appointments. Hunter's complaint was that the surgeon in question, a Mr Hollings, had not been recommended by Hunter, had no experience of army practice and that, 'neither his merit as a man, nor as a surgeon, intitle [*sic*] him to be the cause of such an innovation'.[32] Hunter argued that it was essential that his policy of appointing surgeons who had already seen service with the army be maintained. He noted the experience of those surgeons with military diseases, but most strenuously argued that his recruitment policy, by which he engaged 'young men to enter as mates to Regiments upon the Faith of future promotion', gave those men a right to such appointments. He submitted that if his system were not followed he would lose the confidence he had acquired.

Hunter also initiated an inquiry into the surgical department of the military hospitals with the Duke's armies, and sent his brother-in-law, Everard Home, to investigate.[33] Home did not find any serious problems in the hospitals he visited, however he did encounter significant resistance from Kennedy who did not accept Home's authority. Kennedy told Home outright that he considered himself to be 'acting under the Duke of York without any reference to the Surgeon General, or anyone in England but the Commander in Chief'.[34] Home was made aware of Kennedy's support from the Duke of York, the Duke himself telling Home, 'that the British Troops has [*sic*] suffered very little, and that the different branches of the Hospital Department had been conducted ever since the arrival of the Superintendent General intirely [*sic*] to his satisfaction'.[35] The refusal of the Duke and Kennedy to allow Home any authority in the hospitals was reiterated to him when he attempted to organize the embarkation of invalids at Ostend, and he quickly reached the conclusion that his time on the Continent 'could not materially promote the Service'.[36] He made some minor recommendations with Kennedy's approval, and left.

Kennedy's attitude did not change on the appointment of the new AMB, if anything his claims to autonomy became more strident. Soon after their appointment Keate wrote to Col. St Leger at Head Quarters in Flanders on the pretext that Kennedy had not supplied the name of any place where letters could reach him. He noted Kennedy's recent letter informing Keate of his recommendations of several medical men to His Royal Highness for promotion. In the most restrained terms Keate asked St Leger to communicate to the Duke his and Gunning's commissions empowering them 'to recommend jointly such Physicians, Surgeons and mates belonging either to the Hospital Staff or Regiments, as well abroad as at home as we shall judge to be the most proper'.[37] Keate couched his appeal to the Duke in terms of his desire to comply with the commands of 'his Majesty's positive instructions', and a desire to carry out the grave responsibility of his task. St Leger evidently communicated the contents of Keate's letter to the Duke but it appears that such reasoning carried no weight with him as he gave 'positive and explicit commands' supporting Kennedy's right to recommend medical officers for promotion, and to appoint other men into the vacancies thereby created.[38]

Soon after, Kennedy himself wrote to Gunning in terms that could not have been more inflammatory:

> In the Hospitals here which I have the honour to direct under the Command of HRH the D of York, I have reason to believe that he is perfectly satisfied with all my Arrangements even in the most arduous situations during the campaign ... and as I hold myself responsible for the abilities of those whom I think worthy to recommend to HRH for promotion, I am sedulous in my selection, HRH had given me upon that account his confidence in these matters, and will not permit any interference, I am pretty sure both you and Mr Keate will see this in the light you both did before you were called to the situation in which you are now placed – tho' no Interference is allowed by HRH to take place from home in this Hospital, be assured, Sir, I shall consider myself happy in protecting and providing for your or Mr Keate's Recommendation, knowing well, that I might take the same liberty with you.[39]

Incensed, Keate and Gunning forwarded this message to Lord Amherst and asked for his opinion on such an 'extraordinary' letter that was so 'repugnant to the commands His Majesty was so graciously pleased to give us'.[40] On 1 January 1794, they went even further and made an official complaint about Kennedy's conduct.[41] Happily for them, Amherst confirmed that the King had directed that

all Recommendations of Physicians and Surgeons for the Hospitals, and for the
Medical Staffs Abroad, and at Home, and also of the Surgeons to be appointed to
Regiments, shall be made by the Surgeon General and Inspector of the Regimental
Hospitals, He cannot approve of any recommendation whatever but such as come to
Him agreeably to these Directions.[42]

Gunning then wrote to Kennedy informing him of this order, whilst also communicating in no uncertain terms that he had never been appointed 'Director'
of Hospitals, only being in fact a 'mere inspector', that his commission gave him
no power to recommend any 'Physical person to the Service', and that he had 'no
good judgement … in the Chirurgical line'.[43] The tone of this letter indicates that
Kennedy's activities had severely angered Keate and Gunning.

They also took the step of communicating His Majesty's decision to the medical directors of each of the other expeditions being undertaken by the British at
this time.[44] Additionally, Keate took the precaution of writing to St Leger, telling
him about Gunning's letter to Kennedy and suggesting he read it.[45] Interestingly,
Keate apologized to St Leger for the disturbance this dispute had caused among
the surgeons on the Continent, stating the upset caused to the medical staff was
necessitated by the precedent the decision would set for other campaigns.[46]

However, the AMB were to enjoy only a short-lived victory. Kennedy continued to refuse the yoke of the AMB and the medical staff remained confused
about who was in charge and whether or not they had been promoted. One
young surgeon wrote to his family:

> There have been great abuses in the Medical Establishment here. Mr Keate the Direc-
> tor General at home and Dr. Kennedy the same abroad having been at variance,
> those who are recommended by the former are not attended to by the latter, who,
> though the patronage belongs to Mr Keate, has taken upon him to appoint Hos-
> pital Mates here as he pleases. One consequence has been that four of us here, Day,
> Procter, another and myself, who have had Mr Keate's interest here, have great reason
> to believe we have actually been appointed by him to the staff, though Dr. Kennedy
> has neglected to inform us of it; this circumstance I have mentioned in my letter to
> Mr Keate. I intend also to call upon Dr. Kennedy as soon as I can find him.[47]

Kennedy paid absolutely no attention to the AMB, and continued to act as he
had always done and did so with the apparent backing of the Duke.[48] In addition the AMB now had to face another challenge to their authority, as military
commanders began rejecting their appointments.[49] In a conversation following
one of those rejections, Amherst tactfully communicated the King's desire that
the AMB should respect recommendations from the Duke of York. However,
the AMB did not have the sense to let the matter rest and made further complaints to Amherst. The argument the AMB members presented was supported
in several different ways. In the first instance they asserted the inability of military leaders to make medical staffing decisions: 'no Commander in Chief can

be a judge of Medical or Chirurgical Merit, and must receive his Information through the medium of some Medical Person'. They then returned to their familiar crutch, appealing to the propriety of obedience to His Majesty's commands: 'His Majesty having been pleased to consider the present AMB competent to the Duty reposed in them has not delegated this Trust to any Individual'. Finally, they went on to predict dire consequences if their recommendations were not followed.[50]

The AMB's attempts to find an argument that would appeal to the King were unsuccessful. Amherst answered their letter on the same day stating:

> I have layed [*sic*] before the King your letter to me of this day; His Majesty perused it, but did not give me any particular Orders, I therefore conclude His Majesty did not intend to make any alteration in what he has directed.[51]

While the King may have been willing to endorse the AMB's ascendancy over another medical practitioner, the claims of the Duke were not to be trumped.

Over the course of the Wars, a succession of senior medical officers attempted to assert their independence from the central authority of the AMB. Like Kennedy, those who were successful usually had a powerful military patron. In Kennedy's approach we can also discern that he, like other successful army practitioners, was beginning to pursue medical authority within the army by asserting his expertise, but (unlike the AMB) not at the expense of the authority of military leaders. The claims made by regimental surgeons and their advocates, such as Sinnott and Borland, tied in neatly with this paradigm in which the expertise they asserted was closely linked to the endorsement of military norms like discipline and camaraderie. In contrast, the AMB's naïve and clumsy attempts to use 'military' language, appealing to rigid command structures and transparently flattering the 'humane' intentions of the leaders were unsuccessful.

Challenges to the Army Medical Board

The AMB was also dealing with similar issues at home, where military commanders were attempting to take control of the medical affairs within their purview and senior physicians refused to accept the authority of the surgeon general.

In early 1794, the AMB began receiving troubling reports of a putrid fever in the Hospitals at Chatham, Deal and Plymouth. The AMB took action and sent Dr John Hunter (1754–1809)[52] to Chatham to deal with the problem.[53] Hunter did attend the hospitals, but in early March, Keate had still not received his report and requested it from him. Hunter's response must have questioned Keate's authority to do so, because Keate was forced to write again, outlining the nature of his authority to regulate 'the Conduct & attendance of the different officers in the Hospitals, without which, were there no such Inspection of

Controul [*sic*], the service might suffer'.[54] Hunter held out, and Keate was forced to attend the hospitals himself, but made sure Amherst was aware of it.[55] The matter did not rest there and both parties attempted to involve the secretary at war, Hunter asserting his refusal as a physician to submit to the authority of a mere surgeon, and the AMB advancing the claim that Keate was acting not as a surgeon, but as inspector of hospitals. The professional dispute was augmented with arguments that they hoped would win the sympathy of Amherst:

> [Hunter's] Charging the Inspector, finally, with the attempt to introduce Disorder and to break down all distinction between Ranks in the medical Department is scarcely deserving an Answer. The man who disobeys orders, according to my sphere of understanding is the only person who introduces disorder.[56]

Under the barrage of scorn directed at him by Hunter, Keate also made a plea to the secretary at war to confirm his authority.[57]

It is ironic that the AMB was stymied in the performance of its duties by an objection based on the primacy of physicians over surgeons from a practitioner firmly of the old-school. The incident is representative of the problem many medical practitioners were having at this time: they did not adjust well to the demands of military service and to an extent the military did not know how to incorporate them and their professional sensitivities. It has already been shown that the AMB was floundering in the military environment. At the other end of the scale, Dr Hunter, like Kennedy, reacted badly to any scrutiny of his practice by other practitioners. However, this type of scrutiny was to become an essential feature of military medical practice during the Wars, and men like Hunter were not to ingratiate themselves with military leaders. The difference with Kennedy was that he supported his claim to independence on the expressed wishes of the Duke of York, not merely on a desire to preserve his professional autonomy.

The AMB was not popular with military leaders based near the other hospitals in England either. A site of particular disgruntlement existed in Plymouth where large numbers of recruits were being landed from Cork, the vast majority riddled with fever and many also with dysentery. The commander at Plymouth, Lord George Lennox, wrote repeatedly to the War Office requesting assistance and especially the construction of a general hospital which he believed would help to deal with the growing numbers of sick troops.[58] He was given some assistance by Sir Jerome Fitzpatrick, the inspector of gaols and madhouses in Ireland who had volunteered to accompany the 40th Regiment on their passage from Ireland.[59] Fitzpatrick agreed with Lennox that a proper hospital and quarantine establishment was necessary in Plymouth, and made a strong argument against the embarkation of men in Ireland, where he believed a proper military hospital should also be built. He identified the crowded transports as the most significant contributor to the production of the fever.[60] Despite his advice, the sick continued to arrive at Plymouth and Lennox's letters became increasingly frantic as the crisis continued.[61] Eventually Lennox received a letter from the AMB setting out its opinion of his incompetence to decide whether a hospital was the best solution or not:

> From the letter of Lord George Lennox it appears, that His Lordship is anxious for the immediate erection of an Hospital at Plymouth with a full Medical Establishment. We are ready to pay all proper deference and respect to His Lordship's opinion and Recommendation, but His Lordship will we hope pardon us, if in the execution of our Duty, we doubt whether His Lordship can be fully informed and qualified to judge of such points as require no small degree of experience in medicine and the cure of Diseases, from which to form an accurate judgement.[62]

Lennox's affront at this slight was palpable, especially as no medical aid was actually forthcoming. In December 1794, after more than a year of dealing with the horrendous conditions at Plymouth he wrote:

> I have only to lament that since their letter which was written above seven months ago, we have not experienced any relief; I was in hopes that as it was so clearly pointed out that I could know nothing of the matter, that the Medical Board would have sent some person here that did[63]

In the same letter he equated the mortality rate experienced by the 40th Regiment in Plymouth to a regiment attacked by yellow fever in the West Indies, and indicated that he intended to request a leave of absence at Christmas to get away from 'what I see and can't help'.

Matters on the Continent had not improved either; in June 1794 complaints from some medical officers had prompted the Duke of York to investigate Kennedy's medical arrangements, and Gunning had also made a tour of inspection.[64] However, like Lennox, many military commanders there became increasingly despondent over the medical care being provided to the troops. Colonel Craig wrote to the secretary at war giving his opinion of the medical arrangements organized by Kennedy. The picture he painted was a bleak one:

> It gives me very great concern to say that this department which is so essential is most extremely ill conducted. I know not to whom to attribute it and still less how to remedy it, but I feel for it very much. One great cause of the mismanagement is undoubtedly the spirit of discord which reigns within the department. I am convinced no one member of it will attempt to rectify any thing, the blame of which he imagines will fall upon the shoulders of another man. I declare if I had my wish I would change them all from the first to the last.[65]

By November he reported:

> Our sick list is enormous, very near 7000 which is not very short of one fourth of our number. It is to be hoped that the cold weather will check it. Many of our medical

people are affected by it at the very moment when their services are most wanted, two of the physicians are very dangerously ill and I believe another is incapable of attending his Duty.[66]

The dire straights in which the army found itself, prompted Lt General Harcourt to write to the Duke of York declaring that, 'if something is not decided upon, and very speedily too, the sending of the sick to the general Hospital ... is doing little better than [sending] them to destruction'.[67] Along with General Fox, Lt Colonel Don and Lt Colonel Brownrigg, he had developed a plan for the 'better management of the General Hospital'.[68] This plan, which suggested the formation of a hospital corps to replace the convalescents used as ward masters and orderly men, is especially significant because it was formulated without the input of medical officers and clearly envisaged that significant improvements could be achieved without medical assistance. It provides an excellent demonstration of the medical expertise military leaders perceived themselves to have, largely because of the importance they attributed to discipline and order in the pursuit of a healthy army.

It is not clear what became of Harcourt's plan, but his discontent with the medical arrangements continued, in January he reported:

the bad management of [the Hospitals] I am sorry to say is disgraceful to Great Britain and can never I fear be corrected by the present Director General and Purveyor, who tho' good men, I cannot hesitate in declaring are utterly incapable of performing the duties of their offices.[69]

And in February:

I am sorry to be obliged to repeat that the Three Heads of it Doctors Kennedy, Smyth and Mr Wood the Purveyor though very good men in their private characters have neither abilities, activity, or nerves, even to be of the least use, and that unless others are appointed who are more equal to the task we must despair of ever seeing the least order, attention, or discipline in the Hospital.[70]

Military commanders were seeking senior medical officers in a different shape to that offered by the AMB and the British medical establishment. The shape they were looking for was presented to them in the person of Dr Robert Jackson who was appointed to Kennedy's position after Kennedy's death in April 1795.

Jackson had begun his medical career in 1774 in Jamaica where he first gained experience of military medicine. He also served in America, Flanders and San Domingo, pursuing what he described as his purpose in life, the 'investigation of the physical condition and the moral character of man'.[71] He was particularly preoccupied with the nature of fevers and the practice of army medicine. In 1791 he published his first work on army medicine, focusing on the health of soldiers in hot climates.[72] He was convinced of the importance of the health of soldiers to military success and advocated the prevention of disease with discipline, temperance, exercise, bathing and a simple diet. He also wrote extensively about day-to-day matters such as the location of encampments or stations and appropriate clothing for soldiers. He was a great advocate of bleeding, purging, blistering and shockingly cold baths as therapies for those afflicted with fever. Most of his recommendations were contrary to established military practice but more controversial were his opinions on the structure of the medical department. Jackson was particularly critical of the education of medical recruits. He believed military medicine required specific training and that the examination system in place at the time was no real test of a medical officer's ability. He was also extremely critical of army general hospitals that he regarded as expensive and superfluous hothouses of disease that were ruinous to military discipline.[73]

Jackson had been a surgeon's apprentice, was educated in medicine at Edinburgh but left without a degree, and finally obtained an MD at Leiden in 1785. Accordingly, he was ineligible for the position of army physician and instead had accepted the post of surgeon to the 3rd Regiment of foot. However, his status as a regimental surgeon did not diminish his abilities in the eyes of his military commanders.

In September 1794, Jackson's claims to promotion had been advanced by Lt Colonel Harry Calvert, *aide-de-camp* to the Duke of York,[74] who expressed at the same time his frustrations with the AMB:

> Thank you for ... the trouble you have taken with Jackson. Is it not shameful that a man who is able and willing to render essential service where it is so much wanted should be rejected, or meet with difficulties from a parcel of bigwigs, who, lolling in their chariots in London, call themselves military surgeons, military physicians, and military directors?[75]

He repeated these sentiments in October, when General Balfour appears to have also taken up Jackson's cause: 'I join with General Balfour in urging Dr. Jackson's appointment as physician to this or the West India army. For our own sakes, I wish the former; for the sake of our suffering friends in the west, the Latter'.[76]

Balfour had previously come into conflict with the AMB when it attempted to thwart his preferred appointment of surgeon to his regiment.[77] Jackson's appointment in April as physician to the general hospital at Bremen and as principal medical officer on the Continent has traditionally been attributed to the Duke of York's personal intervention.[78] It is also commonly asserted that the AMB was strongly opposed to Jackson's appointment, and this seems very likely; however, the only reference in the available records is a rather churlish one made in June 1795.[79] Jackson's exertions in this role were applauded by his military commanders[80] and he was specifically exempted from complaints made by military officers about the medical arrangements after the campaign.[81]

Jackson was to become an archetype held up by advocates of a military medical speciality throughout the course of the Wars, and the events of the Low Countries campaign involving him were used frequently in arguments against the recruitment and promotions policy of the AMB.[82]

The AMB continued to face military resistance to their authority, and commanders in Corsica, the West Indies and the East Indies constantly attempted to appoint their own medical officers.[83] Sir Ralph Abercrombie insisted on taking Dr Thomas Young with him to the Leeward Isles, dismissing the AMB-appointed inspector, Dr Macdonald.[84] Young, in turn, informed the AMB that he would be making his own promotions and sent home the hospital mates appointed by the AMB.[85] In the face of this opposition, the AMB continued to make arguments for their own expertise in the selection of medical officers, but in doing so further alienated the military establishment:

> the Appointment of Medical Persons must turn in propriety on Three points; that of Length of Service, Ability or an overruling necessity ... though Commanders in chief may judge as well as others upon the first and third qualifications they are not competent to judge on the second, and that His Majesty has Delegated that to others, for that purpose.[86]

> For it is impossible that Medical Knowledge or merit can be judged of but by Medical Men. It is a Constant Observation that a Physician Practices his Profession, *coram non judice*, whereas in other professions the world are judges of merit and knowledge.[87]

It is perhaps for this reason that the AMB's more palatable arguments regarding the importance of adherence to rank and expectation in the maintenance of goodwill among junior medical officers, and concerns about the quality of care given to His Majesty's deserving troops fell on deaf ears.

In the first ten years of the Wars, military officers became quickly disillusioned with the services provided by AMB-appointed medical officers, and rejected AMB arguments that military commanders were unable to judge the abilities of medical officers for themselves. Medical officers keen to establish their careers outside the narrow and hierarchical paths allowed by the AMB quickly saw that it was essential to adopt a distinctly 'military' approach, and incorporated discipline and respect for military command structures and patronage networks into their practices.

Disease Theory and 'Military Diseases'

The ongoing insistence of the AMB on the primacy of civilian-based Oxbridge training was an important factor underlying the newly forming articulation of a separate professional identity for military medical officers. Another factor that contributed to it was an increasing incidence of encounters with epidemics and diseases that were substantially different to anything these practitioners had learned about in lectures and classic medical texts, or seen in civilian practice.

It is well established that medical officers serving in the West Indies in the decade prior to 1800 developed a distinct approach to medicine that favoured observation and experiment.[88] Environmental conceptions of disease, bloodletting, cold-water therapies and a tendency towards anticontagionism in respect to yellow fever were also common in their practices. The diseases of the West Indies were characterized as 'tropical diseases' and many medical men had thought for some time that they were different in important respects to the diseases of a British climate.[89] The experiences of military medical officers in the Low Countries, and in the West Indian campaigns which followed, led many to the conclusion that 'military diseases' also constituted a separate category of disease, and that additionally there was something special about the doctors that treated them.

Following the Low Countries campaigns, several publications appeared which discussed the deficiencies of the medical arrangements that had been made for the army.[90] Such works also considered the nature of the fever that had ravaged the troops as well as its likely causes. The most significant of these was Robert Jackson's *Outline of the History and Cure of Fever*. In this work, which is primarily devoted to his experiences in the West Indies, Jackson gave a medical history of the British army in Holland over the retreat of 1794–5. Jackson characterized the fever as contagious and brought about by 'artificial causes'. By this he meant that the fever was not the endemic fever of the Low Countries, but instead was brought about by the behaviour and management of the troops. He argued that it was introduced by the recruitment of unfit men, 'rendered virulent by accumulation in General Hospitals', and propagated and diffused by poor discipline and arrangement.[91] His implication, that the fever would not have been able to take such a hold on the army if it had been comprised of fit and virtuous men who were well commanded and kept under a proper discipline, intimately associated the disease with the constitution of the army, and its cure with military values. Previous discussions of disease and the army had focused on the relationship of the troops with their natural environment, and largely attributed the diseases they encountered to the foreign environments in which armies often operated.[92] Although Jackson's representation of the 1794–5 fever resonates with discussions about order, discipline and disease amongst seamen at this time,[93] his characterization of the army *as* the disease differs in that the fever is specific to the military, and thus a 'military disease'.[94] Jackson took the concept further later in his argument and described the specific modes of fever that were particular to the various types of army organization.

Jackson's identification of the lack of discipline in the army as a direct cause of the fever is echoed in the writings of other practitioners who served on these campaigns. Borland identified 'feeble discipline' an important proximate cause of the epidemic, but focused more on the role of the general hospitals and 'accumulation' in the transformation of the fever into a contagion, which then disseminated throughout the army. William Fergusson and James McGrigor, both of whom were in the formative stages of their military medical careers at this time, also stressed these elements regarding the cause of the fever. All these men emerged from the campaign with a strong antipathy to general hospitals, which they believed did not only make existing diseases worse through 'accumulation', but actually caused disease in the army.[95] As will be demonstrated in the following chapter, this was to have a significant impact on the development of military medicine and the 'military medical officer' identity.

The experience acquired by practitioners serving on these campaigns was also seen by them as conferring an expertise that could not be achieved in civilian practice. Writing just after the Wars, Fergusson commented that the campaign of 1794 had enabled him to compare his learning about typhus and hospital practice with the reality of an epidemic. He believed that he had gathered 'materials for reflection' about the disease that 'bore a stamp which nothing in the medical practice of a civil life could have impressed'. He also asserted that he had seen more cases of typhus there than he would have seen in Edinburgh over the course of an entire civilian career.[96] Fergusson bolstered his claims in this regard with reference to his service in the West Indies: 'But if this impression had not been sufficiently strong, I had next, in the years 1796, 1797, and 1798, to perform the duties of a surgeon ... under the still more destructive scourge of the yellow fever, in St Domingo'.[97]

The West Indies were an important theatre during the first ten years of the Wars, and campaigns were waged for control of the lucrative islands from April 1793, when Britain launched a minor attack on the French garrison of Tobago. More significant were the struggle for control of St Domingo, beginning in June 1794, a series of French backed rebellions against the British in the Windward Isles in 1795, and the British offensive to recapture them in 1796. These campaigns coincided with a particularly virulent outbreak of yellow fever amongst the European troops, putting enormous strain on the medical officers many of whom believed they were encountering a new disease. Estimates of the losses from disease vary, but the most recent scholarly estimate of approximately 15,000 men appears to be the most accurate.[98] There were many important developments in medicine that sprang from these campaigns,[99] but for the purposes of this book only those that relate to the growing articulation of a military medical specialty will be considered.

As indicated by Fergusson above, many practitioners who had been inducted into military service in the Low Countries were next sent out to the Caribbean. They were confronted with what appeared to be a new disease, and many were led to question received learning about the nature of such fevers, particularly the doctrine that they were contagious: 'All, I may say, came out contagionists, myself amongst the number, none remained so'.[100] Additionally, new or resurrected therapeutics were advocated amongst these practitioners – including such bold measures as cold water dousing, bloodletting and blistering.[101] These treatments were promoted by Jackson,[102] and his work was referred to extensively by other military medical men serving in the Caribbean.

Hector McLean was one of Jackson's admirers. In 1798, he published his own account of the epidemic in which he advocated a similar approach to the treatment of the disease.[103] McLean specifically addressed his book to the army.[104] Like Jackson, McLean identified aspects of military discipline that could help prevent or control the disease, but he also expressly referred to the position of the medical officer in the army, alleging that without the support of a commanding officer, medical officers could do very little. In this way, McLean asserted his perception of the relationship between military authority and the preservation of health – embedding effective military medicine firmly within military organization.[105] McLean also made claims for the specialized knowledge required to treat military diseases, knowledge that could only be acquired on service:

> It is absurd to send out physicians from London, to combat the diseases of St Domingo – the requisite knowledge for this purpose can only be acquired on the spot, after a long, painful, and accurate attention ...
> Those who have followed the army and acquired experience, are inestimable.[106]

McLean reasoned that army practitioners not only had the necessary understanding of the diseases they faced, but also most importantly understood the habits and manners of soldiers. Similarly, William Lempriere (although a much more conventional practitioner) believed that the treatment of soldiers in the West Indies required specialized knowledge that could only be gleaned through experience and endeavoured to pass on the wisdom he had acquired during these campaigns to young regimental surgeons.[107]

By the end of the campaigns in the Low Countries and the Caribbean, young military medical officers had encountered disease in forms and virulence for which their education and training had not prepared them. This led them to question received learning about diseases and to posit that there was much not accounted for in classic medical texts. They began to argue that distinct 'military diseases' existed, and that those diseases required specialized training and experience. They also began to support therapeutics not known, or out of fashion in civilian medical circles, and to develop new ones based on their observations on campaigns. Many of their recommendations for prevention and cure were intimately related to military discipline and order, and accordingly helped to form a distinct military medical vocabulary.

Conclusion

During the first ten years of the Wars, military medical officers were exposed to a number of factors that caused them to re-evaluate their professional identities and to assert the contribution they were making to the British army. The criticism of their education, training and experience was set up in direct contrast to an Oxbridge medical education, and forced men grounded in the former career path to consider how they could justify their entitlements to promotion and to professional respect. Combined with the developments in disease theory that resulted from these campaigns, this reconsideration resulted in the emerging concepts of 'military disease' and a specialized 'military medicine'. The unwillingness of some senior military practitioners to submit themselves to the authority of the AMB prompted them to cultivate the patronage of senior military officers by incorporating military values such as discipline and regimental bonds into their schemes for the preservation of health, and by appealing to military values in the rhetoric they employed. In order to achieve medical success within the army, it was essential not only to be relatively successful in curing patients, but also to 'talk the military talk', and not to minimize or dismiss the contribution of military commanders and military norms to that process. In the letters of military commanders, we can see how they perceived the relationship between military and medical needs and why men like those on the AMB, and physicians wedded to privilege like Hunter, were gradually to lose the battle to define the course of British military medicine as the Wars progressed.

2 WALCHEREN AND THE ARMY MEDICAL BOARD

The AMB was overhauled again in 1798 and given a new constitution. Sir Lucas Pepys and Thomas Keate remained on the AMB as physician and surgeon general, respectively, and Francis Knight was appointed inspector general of army hospitals. The AMB's new constitution divided previously shared responsibilities, created overlapping duties and resulted in illogical processes of appointment and promotion of medical officers.[1] The Board was notorious for the infighting in which its members engaged and it was eventually discontinued. On 27 February 1810, the *London Gazette* announced the appointment of John Weir as director general and Theodore Gordon and Charles Kerr as principal inspectors of a new board 'for superintending and conducting the whole Medical Business of the Army'.

The divisions within the AMD, between the AMB and the new school of 'military medical officers' adverted to in Chapter 1, widened during the course of the 1798 Board's tenure and provided a key focus for the expression of competing visions of the future of the AMD and military medicine generally. This chapter will examine those conflicts, which culminated in an inquiry into the Walcheren Campaign in 1809. It will show that debates about military medicine became violently personal and factionalized and that the vicious nature of these debates was driven not solely by an intellectual commitment to particular theories of disease, but also by a desire to procure the patronage of powerful men, such as the members of the AMB. It is plausible that this desire for patronage even contributed to the medical philosophy and therapeutic choices made by many medical practitioners, particularly new medical recruits. It will also be demonstrated that while the men at the forefront of these debates were apparently arguing about appropriate medical practice, in fact they were striving to assert and control competing visions of the future of the medical profession: a future in which they perceived there would be a limited market for medical services. Ironically, the ultimate effect of these debates was the erosion of military medicine's professional autonomy as government was forced to step in and, in effect, decide medical debates.

The Walcheren Campaign

Rifleman Harris described the horrors of the Walcheren campaign as follows:

> The company I belonged to was quartered in a barn, and I quickly perceived that hardly a man there had stomach for the bread that was served out to him, or even to taste his grog ... about three weeks from the day we landed, I and two others were the only individuals who could stand upon our legs. They lay groaning in rows in the barn, amongst the heaps of lumpy black bread they were unable to eat.[2]

It was a campaign notable for its size, the 'peculiarity that there was not one naval or military officer who had given their sanction to the project',[3] and the spectacular devastation wrought by disease among the British troops.[4] More than 40,000 British troops aboard hundreds of vessels, including thirty-three ships of the line, set sail in July 1809 for the island of Walcheren off the Zeeland coast of the Netherlands.[5] The expedition was intended to support the Fifth Coalition's land campaign by securing the islands of the Scheldt, destroying the enemy's naval force in that river, cutting off enemy resources at Antwerp and rendering the river impassable to ships of war. None of these objectives was achieved. The monumental failure of the operation was compounded by the loss of nearly 4,000 soldiers to 'Walcheren Fever' and the long-term incapacitation of a further 11,500.[6]

The expedition, commanded by Lord Chatham, arrived at Walcheren on 28 July 1809. From the beginning poor weather conditions hampered operations, disembarkation was delayed and once onshore troops had to contend with constant rain and the already marshy land. In mid-August, sickness appeared spreading with alarming ferocity and by 27 August the sick comprised 3,467 rank and file.[7] On that day a joint military council determined that 'the undertaking of the siege of Antwerp was impracticable' and recommended the operation be terminated.[8] However, it was not until 16 December that the withdrawal and evacuation of sick troops from Walcheren was complete.

The failure of the expedition to the Scheldt was seized upon by the opposition and the entire operation examined in exhaustive detail by a House of Commons inquiry in 1810. The principal targets of the inquisitors were the ministerial architects of the expedition, particularly for their incompetent planning and failure to take into account the (almost unanimous) military and specialist advice against the operation that they had received.

The appalling levels of sickness and death on the expedition ensured that members of the AMB and medical officers who had been at Walcheren were questioned extensively during the inquiry. The evidence given to the House established that the island of Walcheren was notoriously unhealthy, particularly at the time of year in which the expedition was undertaken and that, had they been consulted, the Board members would have advised the government of that fact. However, the Board members demonstrated that they were not consulted until the sickness was well established and, consequently, that the failure to adequately provision the expedition with medical staff and supplies was not their fault.[9] Accordingly, despite the devastating mortality rate, ongoing invalidism of surviving Walcheren troops, and the feuds and unprofessional behaviour of the Board members revealed during the inquiry, the Board was not censured in the inquiry's resolutions.[10]

However, the Walcheren crisis has been seen by many historians as a watershed in the history of the AMD and a significant cause of the AMB's dismissal in February 1810.[11] Arnold Chaplin and Kate Elizabeth Crowe point out that in fact the reconstitution of the Board had been in process since the publication of the 'Fifth Report of the Commissioners of Military Enquiry' in 1808 which found that,

> the offices of Physician General, Surgeon General, Inspector General of Army Hospitals and Comptroller of Army Hospital Accounts should be discontinued, and that the superintendence of the Medical Department of the Army should be placed in a Board of Commissioners, constituted of a Chairman and of two junior Members ... a Board so constituted would, we think, produce much beneficial improvement in the Medical System of the Army.[12]

A review of government correspondence following the publication of the 'Fifth Report' supports Chaplin and Crowe's argument, and demonstrates that the slow wheels of administrative reform were, indeed, turning throughout the two years leading up to the Walcheren inquiry.[13] However, it is generally agreed by all historians that the behaviour of the Board during the Walcheren expedition resulting from their bitter feuds at the very least focused the attention of government on the need for urgent reform.

Very few of the historians who have considered Walcheren have done more than describe the onset of the medical emergency on the island, the ineffective response of the AMB, and the Commons inquiry. None consider the reasons behind the frictions in the Board or the effects of the feuds on the development of military medicine. To undertake that analysis it is necessary to examine the development of those feuds over the course of the Board's tenure. Additionally, the various government inquiries into the operations of the AMD prompted by those feuds, of which the Walcheren Enquiry was merely the last in a long line, must be considered as a whole.

Early Inquiries

Agitation for reform of the AMD had begun in the 1790s, following the failures of the campaigns in the Low Countries. These tracts often referred directly to the specialized nature of military medical practice. Sinnott's 1796 observations on the mismanagement of the AMD and the 'appalling' state of army general hospitals, had also discussed the failure of the service to attract and provide medical men with the requisite skills and knowledge for military practice.[14] A surgeon, John Bell, expressed similar sentiments when in 1800 he called for the establishment of a national school of surgery and anatomy for aspirants to the military medical service focusing on what he perceived to be essential skills for the practice including knowledge of gunshot wounds and medical geography.[15]

The most vocal campaigner for reform in this early period was Robert Jackson. As has been shown, he was brought into direct conflict with the AMB in 1793 when he was given the position of army physician against the Board's recommendation. Very shortly afterwards Jackson's rank was raised to that of inspector of hospitals, again against the advice of the AMB. His rapid and unorthodox promotions earned him the unending enmity of Lucas Pepys and the likeminded surgeon general, Thomas Keate.[16]

Sir Lucas Pepys had a strong and traditional vision of medicine. He did not believe that military medicine required specialized knowledge. He was a firm believer in the importance of the principles of medicine learned at Oxford and Cambridge and pursued a deliberate programme to improve the army medical service, as he saw it, by taking over the department with 'College' men, thus stemming the tide of 'poorly educated' apprentices, come surgeons, come physicians, many of whom had studied at Edinburgh and whom he considered ill-educated pretenders.[17]

Jackson's promotions saw him given charge of the hospital at the military depot on the Isle of Wight. There he implemented his plan for a well-organized army hospital. He insisted on employing his long-term associate, Dr James Borland, to assist him. He arranged the sick into wards according to their illnesses, instituted new (and much reduced) diet tables and pursued his particular forms of therapy, including prolific bleeding and hot bathing followed by immersion in extremely cold water.[18] Jackson appears to have been a proud man with little patience for practitioners who disagreed with him and he deliberately excluded a more traditional colleague at the hospital by ensuring that he had no patients in his wards. The disaffected colleague, Dr Maclaurin, wrote to the AMB about Jackson's practices and the issue was immediately seized upon by Pepys and Keate who saw their chance to bring down the renegade. On 10 December 1801, they wrote to the secretary at war regarding the economy of Jackson's hospital, stating that his methods were the cause of an 'unprecedented number of deaths ... frequent relapses and tedious recoveries', and urging that he should be made to comply with the printed regulations for general hospitals.[19]

Pepys and Keate also obtained letters of evidence from other medical workers at the hospital at Chatham where Jackson and the depot had previously been located. Their complaint resulted in the first of a series of government inquiries into army medical practice and deeply entrenched the animosity between the parties.

The inquiry, conducted by Dr John Hunter, Dr George Pinckard, John Weir and Sir John Macnamara Hayes, found that Jackson's practices, while unorthodox, were not improper and that, conversely, it was appropriate for him to experiment with potentially life-saving innovations.[20] They did recommend that he revise some of his diet tables to be more in line with army guidelines[21] but attributed the high mortality rate to overcrowding of the hospitals and their poor design. The tone of their commendation for Jackson – 'We feel ourselves called upon, in justice, to say, that Dr Jackson appeared to us a zealous, diligent, and meritorious servant of the public, and full of humanity in the discharge of his duty'[22] – indicates that they may have felt the entire inquiry was inappropriate as does their criticism of Keate and Pepys:

> We cannot help thinking that the Army Medical Board have not sufficiently adverted to the mischievous effects of various kinds that must arise from applications to officers in inferior stations for their opinion and judgement of their superiors ... We would recommend, that instead of such proceeding, if the increase of sickness or mortality, or any other causes, shall give rise to suspicion, that the Physician General, or Surgeon General, or both, according to the nature of the case, should themselves investigate the matter on the spot, as the surest means of finding a remedy for the evil.[23]

It is also clear, from the text of this criticism, that they endorsed a view of military medicine in which subordination and discipline according to traditional army notions of hierarchy were applicable to medical officers in the exercise of their clinical judgement. The inquiry can certainly be seen as a victory for Jackson and for his medical views. Nevertheless, following the inquiry Jackson felt he could no longer serve under Pepys and Keate and tendered his resignation.

Despite his resignation from the AMD, Jackson continued to be a thorn in its side. He published several books setting out his views on the proper organization of armies and army medical departments, which developed his 1791 work.[24] These works were more openly critical of the administration of the AMD and were read widely within army circles.[25] One of the themes constantly stressed by Jackson was the superfluity and expense of the general hospital and the importance of conducting even regimental hospitals on more 'economical' principles. Jackson was, however, careful to exclude one member of the AMB, Francis Knight, from his attack. Knight had been appointed in 1801, and was sympathetic to Jackson's view of economical medicine. Knight had served as a surgeon with the Coldstream Guards, and there is no record of his holding a university degree.[26] He agreed with Jackson's assessment of the respective merits of general and regimental hospitals and took it upon himself to shut down most of the general hospitals in England after his appointment.

Knight's appointment saw the emergence of a devastating power struggle within the AMD between the conservative Pepys–Keate coalition and the newcomer who allied himself with Jackson, Borland, and Dr James McGrigor. In addition to his affiliation with Jackson's style of medicine, Knight appears also to have been a difficult and aggressive individual. The inability of the three men to work together soon became notorious and events during and after the 'Fifth Report' made it clear the AMB was untenable.[27]

The 'Fifth Report' and the Debate over General Hospitals

An overriding theme in Jackson's work was extravagance and unnecessary expense in the running of the AMD. Not surprisingly then, when the demands of Spencer Perceval and the Treasury prompted a series of inquiries into the running of the army, the appointed Commissioners of Military Enquiry gave ample consideration to Jackson's views.

Ostensibly, the Commissioners of Military Enquiry were only to examine 'the Public Expenditure, and Conduct of Public Business' in various military departments.[28] However, their investigation of the AMD was significantly wider ranging. They considered not only the constitution and operation of the AMB, but also its system of promotions (including the existence of corruption and bribery), the debate over general versus regimental hospitals and the qualifications of army medical officers. These issues went to the heart of the conflict between men like Pepys who wanted to maintain the privilege and dominance of the College of Physicians in all areas of the profession, and newcomers like Jackson who envisaged a more inclusive profession, open to new ideas, rewarding experience rather than theoretical education.

The debate over general and regimental hospitals that was aired during this inquiry continued throughout the Wars, as did questions over the derivative issue of whether military medicine required specialized knowledge. Accordingly, it is necessary briefly to outline the arguments that were used for and against general hospitals, which changed very little as the debate evolved.

General hospitals were large institutions either in Britain or at the front but well back from the line of battle; they were permanent and unmoving and received men from any regiment for treatment. Regimental hospitals were much smaller, catered principally only to the men of that regiment and were not permanent, moving with the troops. Jackson's arguments against the general hospital were representative of the anti-general hospital party. They were grounded in the idea that general hospitals were too expensive. Jackson argued that general hospitals employed too many staff, wasted food and medical supplies, and often lay idle without patients. He was more strongly opposed to their use overseas than in Britain. In addition, he argued that these hospitals were usually poorly constructed and sited for the promotion of health, and that instead they encouraged the development and spread of disease. He also believed that they were ruinous to the military health of the soldier, the lack of regimental discipline and camaraderie causing the soldier to lose his zest for war and consequently to feign illness in an attempt to stay out of service. One of the reasons regimental hospitals achieved better results, he argued, was that the regimental surgeon knew his patients' constitutions intimately, and had an increased motivation to get them back on their feet.[29]

The opposing party was often reduced to simple denials of all these accusations. Their positive case in defence of the general hospital was usually that, even although they often lay idle, general hospitals provided a critical resource during times of medical crisis. They defended the disparity in mortality rates between the two types of hospital by stating that general hospitals were intended to receive the seriously ill and wounded, as opposed to regimental institutions that were required to send on those patients when the regiment moved forward.[30]

An intrinsic element of the debate related to the type of medical officer that staffed each type of hospital. Regimental hospitals were staffed by 'regimental surgeons'. These men (often Scots who had studied at Edinburgh) typically had received a brief education in medicine before joining a regiment and learning their trade 'on-the-field'. Men like Jackson argued that without this on-the-ground experience of the casualties of war no medical officer could adequately perform military medicine – making the argument for military medicine as a medical speciality.[31] One of the more controversial aspects of this claim was that 'military medicine' blurred the lines between physic and surgery, as regimental surgeons claimed to perform both. Advocates of general hospitals were aware that general hospitals provided employment for physicians and other medical officers who had often not had the experience of serving with a regiment and whose knowledge of medicine had largely been acquired in universities and civilian practice. They argued that military service did not produce diseases different to civilian life, and that without a knowledge of the medical principles acquired in traditional medical education, regimental surgeons were little more than tradesmen patching up the wounded, or worse, conducting ill-conceived 'empirical' experiments not guided by a sound understanding of the human body.[32]

In later years, it became obvious even to some of the most strident participants in this debate that both types of institution served an important purpose.[33] Despite the genuine aversion to general hospitals many medical officers had developed in the Low Countries campaigns, the polarity of the debate must have resulted, in part at least, from self-interest. Men like Pepys sought to maintain their own position and defend the status of physicians above 'persons of inferior medical education'[34] (i.e. deputy inspectors who, under Knight's innovations were higher in authority than physicians). Jackson, representative of the hundreds of medical recruits in this period, attempted to substantiate his own career pathway as a respectable, financially rewarding, and most of all, status bestowing one.[35]

These issues were canvassed widely during the investigation of the Commissioners of Military Enquiry. The commissioners took evidence from, *inter alia*, Pepys, Keate and Knight. They compared the AMD with the equivalent establishments in the Navy, Ordnance, and the East India Company. Significantly, they also took evidence on the AMD from Borland and McGrigor, particularly in relation to regimental and general hospitals. Their evidence prompted the following statement from the commissioners:

> The concurring testimony of these Gentlemen justifies us, we think, in alluding to two publications of Doctor Jackson, who was also a Regimental Surgeon serving at the same period on the Continent, and which state the same facts.[36]

In fact, the commissioners were heavily influenced by Jackson (who lived too far away to be consulted in person), referring to his publications constantly in their report and relying on his opinions.[37]

Their investigation of medical practice was supportive of Jackson. As stated above the commissioners recommended the abolition of the current AMB. They also supported the philosophy of military medicine as a speciality distinct from civilian physic and surgery, thus bestowing a higher value on the experience of regimental and staff surgeons than on the education of the Oxbridge physician:

> When it is considered how peculiar are the manners, the habits, and often even the diseases of the Military, it seems if ... Physicians were necessary in the Army, that there would have been a convenience in selecting them from amongst those Regimental and Staff Surgeons who possessed actual experience in Army Medical practice, both at home and abroad.[38]

They recommended that general hospitals only be used where necessary abroad and not at all domestically[39] and agreed with Jackson that stations abroad comprised too many medical staff.[40]

The report's endorsement of military medicine as a speciality and its adoption of nearly all Jackson's recommendations represented a significant blow to the position of Pepys and Keate (Keate was doubly chastised by the commissioners in their consideration of the AMD's spending).[41] Pepys and Keate were incensed by the report that highlighted their lack of military experience. By recommending men with military experience to run the department, the report profoundly devalued their expertise and education in terms of military service.

The report precipitated a violent escalation in the disputes of the AMB. It was fought in the public sphere through a pamphlet war, the halls of government through appeals to ministers, and even in the streets where in 1809, Jackson attacked Keate with a golden-headed cane. The dispute revealed itself to be about more than medicine as questions about patronage, alliances and education came to the fore. The removal of the dispute to these forums aroused public and government concern. The 'Fifth Report' was criticized by the Pepys/Keate camp for venturing into an arena which only experts (i.e. medical practitioners) could understand, and in considering the way forward, government responded by seeking the expert advice of the AMB. However, the AMB was hamstrung by its dispute. Their inability to advise government, their appeals to ministers for adjudication of their disputes, and the bizarre, churlish behaviour they exhibited during inquiries that followed had the result that, ultimately, it was not medical men who determined the shape of the AMD.

The Pamphlet War

The pamphlet war that followed the 'Fifth Report' was conducted by Keate and Edward Bancroft on one side, and McGrigor, Borland and Jackson on the other. While the findings of the 'Fifth Report' were ostensibly the issues over which they fought, the pamphlets reveal more about the non-medical reasons for their hostility. The issue to emerge most strongly from the pamphlets was the mutual antipathy between advocates of the Oxbridge and Scottish/empirical educational models.

The first response to the 'Fifth Report' was issued by Keate, whose financial management of the AMD had been scathingly criticized.[42] Leaving aside his response to accusations of financial mismanagement, Keate's *Observations* addressed the 'matters of principle' disputed by the two camps: the respective merits of general and regimental hospitals, of army surgeons and College physicians, and the related issue of whether a superfluity of medical staff existed on overseas missions. He also considered the evidence presented regarding other military medical departments and distinguished their circumstances from those facing the army. However, Keate did not restrict his observations to 'matters of principle' and devoted much of his work to character assassinations of those he believed to be responsible for misguiding the commissioners.

Keate took particular offence at the commissioners' decision to

> seek *viva-voce* evidence from two gentlemen only, who certainly were among the least qualified ... since one of them, Dr McGrigor, has never in the whole course of his service been called upon ... to do one day's duty in general hospitals, and the other Dr Borland, has done but little duty in them.[43]

Keate continued to criticize Borland's veracity, expertise and capacity to testify for several pages.[44] He also attempted to discredit McGrigor by questioning the truthfulness of his evidence,[45] and took a similar approach when rebutting the evidence of Mr Young.[46] Keate reserved his most vitriolic attack for Jackson. He stated that Jackson's evidence regarding hospitals in the West Indies was 'an assertion so repugnant to facts ... [that] may naturally create suspicion and a desire of some explanation, especially as so great a part of the report of the Commissioners is founded upon that gentleman's publications'.[47] Keate attached appendices to his pamphlet detailing 'what [Jackson] is capable of doing'[48] to those who disagreed with him (referring to a legal dispute in the West Indies), and one going into depth on the incidents at the Isle of Wight (from Keate's perspective).

In addition to making serious personal allegations, Keate constantly criticized these men for their lack of education. He stated that

> it must still be confessed, that Staff Officers, whether Physicians or Surgeons, who are selected on account of superior education ... are more likely to bring about the speedy recovery of their patients in General Hospitals than could be expected ... in Regimental Hospitals.[49]

He alleged that most who obtained a degree in medicine from a Scotch university, had paid for it without taking any examination.[50]

Borland was quick to answer Keate's publication.[51] In a letter addressed to the inspector general of army hospitals, he voiced his outrage that Keate has 'more than insinuate[d] that little credit is to be given to my evidence on oath, as having misrepresented facts'.[52] Responding to the slights on his education, he made much of the value of experience, 'I do not yield to the Surgeon General, for he never served as a Staff Surgeon with armies, or performed operations in the field'.[53]

Jackson also responded to Keate in two letters, one addressed directly to him[54], and one to the Commissioners of Military Enquiry.[55] The letter to Keate is an exhaustive, self-righteous, consideration of the Isle of Wight affair. The second letter is of more relevance to this discussion. In it Jackson expanded on his views of general hospitals and the arrangement of the medical service in the West Indies, he also defended his expertise based on experience and the importance of experiment.[56]

The pamphlet war reached higher levels of name-calling (and lower pretensions to actual debate) when Bancroft joined the fray. Although he had served on several campaigns with the army, Dr Bancroft was a Cambridge man and very much of the 'old school'.[57] He was a close ally of Pepys and Keate.[58] His *Letter to the Commissioners of Military Enquiry* is deeply critical of the commissioners' decision to rely on the:

> publications of a writer, noted for a strong propensity to innovating projects and speculations, as well as for eccentric and peculiar opinions, and who from the course and events of his life, must have adopted lasting prejudices on several topics to which that inquiry was directed.[59]

In it he conceded the value of experience in medicine but adhered to Pepys's claim that a 'knowledge of principles' was more important, for without it 'experience is generally useless, and frequently delusive, at best it could produce only a mechanical or empirical routine of practice'.[60] He asserted the superiority of civilian practitioners over regimental[61] and further degraded the importance of military experience by stating that there were no such things as distinct 'Army Medical Practice' or military diseases.[62] His personal attacks on McGregor [*sic*],[63] William Yates[64] and Francis Knight,[65] questioned their professional competence. His particular criticism, however, was of regimental surgeons in general. He asserted:

> *physicians* are qualified *above all other men* by means which education has afforded them, of taking comprehensive views of the diseases most frequently prevalent in different climates and situations, of the causes of such diseases, and of the best modes of obviating them[66]

He further commented upon the commissioners' recommendation to exclude physicians from the army, stating that it would make Britain appear to prefer 'an uninformed, unprincipled empiricism in the treatment of those who may want medical assistance'.[67]

Bancroft's pamphlet drew an outraged response from McGrigor. McGrigor's *Letter to the Commissioners of Military Enquiry*[68] evidences both his affiliation with Knight and an attempt to curry favour with him, 'Your investigation began at a time, when, by the indefatigable industry, and incorruptible integrity of one individual, an effectual remedy had been applied to most of the abuses which had previous existed'.[69] McGrigor's response to Bancroft's accusations of untruthfulness under oath supports Shapin's argument about the importance of truthfulness to the concept of gentlemanly identity, and demonstrates that it remained relevant during the eighteenth century.[70] McGrigor perceived such an attack to be the 'vilest of all charges'[71] and claimed, 'In independence of spirit, if not of fortune, I will not yield to him, or to any man'.[72] The severity of the accusation is reflected in the tone of McGrigor's direct challenge to Bancroft:

> Away with such dark and assassin-like insinuations. Speak out like a man, I am fully prepared to meet you ... And to compel you, if possible, to accept this challenge, I thus publicly declare, that, unless you do speak out, I shall regard you in no better light, than that of a malignant and dastardly assassin.[73]

Jackson's response was milder. Perhaps used to such accusations, he gave them little notice, once again devoting his attention to the merits of the regimental surgeon. In uncharacteristic style, he set out his position very plainly. He conceded that the regimental surgeon is 'often obscure in rise, and irregular in progress' but then made the clear statement that he trusted 'no other qualification except possession of the knowledge of [his] profession'.[74] He railed against Pepys and the exclusion of the military surgeon from the post of physician. True to his empiricist philosophy, he challenged Pepys to a bizarre experiment to determine the better style of medicine. His proposal was to give half a regiment to him alone to care for and the other half to Pepys. Death rates would decide the matter. His challenge was not taken seriously.

Unwilling to let the matter rest, Bancroft replied to both Jackson and McGrigor.[75] In this, the most childish of all the letters, Bancroft suggested that McGrigor did not know how to spell his own name, asserted that he would no longer refer to Borland as 'Dr' but only as 'Mr' (since his qualifications could not be proved), and that Jackson could neither read nor write. These accusations graphically illustrate that a very important aspect of the regimental versus general hospital debate following the 'Fifth Report' was the quality of education of the practitioners who staffed them. The issue directly touched on the competence of the medical practitioners of those institutions, giving the debate a very personal quality as both groups attempted to assert the superiority of their education, both for military practice and as medical practitioners more generally.

The medical community was, at this time, very aware of the much-reduced availability of military medical positions and likely flooding of the civilian British medical market upon the cessation of war. The Peace of Amiens in 1802 had provided a small taste of what peace would bring. The debate over general and regimental hospitals should be viewed in this context, and the avowals of the protagonists in favour of one or the other also seen partially as an affirmation of their right to employment in the post-war market. One medical commentator had previously characterized the Oxbridge doctors thus:

> You are afraid of these practical men; hence arises your tenacity: you are afraid of being placed on a superannuated list; a list many of you would handsomely decorate. You behold in perspective, these Scotch graduates sitting at the table you once sat at, enjoying the most exquisite dainties, as a reward of their practical knowledge, while the theoretic knowledge of an Oxford or Cambridge graduate, scarcely can procure a common subsistence.[76]

While medical officers certainly had an eye on future employment, they were also firmly focused on present advancement within the military and, according to the practice of the time, were mindful of the requirements of patronage – those in power wanted to cultivate their personal empires, and those looking for advancement wanted the patronage of great men. An anonymous author wrote about the relevance of these considerations in his review of the above pamphlets:

> I do not pretend to know whether Mr Keate's predilection in favour of general hospitals be founded on unbiased opinion, or a sense of their utility in a view of patronage ...

Their dispute respecting general and regimental hospitals, as I have before remarked, seems always to have been conducted in the spirit of party ... The contest respecting the two kinds of hospitals, indeed, appears to have been chiefly for patronage, and it also appears that Mr Knight and the regimental hospitals have prevailed.[77]

W. M. Nisbet in his analysis of the 'Fifth Report' made the telling comment:

Thus the pretended abuses and faults, pointed out by the Report of the Military Commission, are nothing more than the desire of each individual to extend the powers of his own department, and to give it as much importance as possible, being the means of increasing his own influence, his own consequence, and his own reputation.[78]

These commentaries must give pause to any historian who is tempted to take the debate over general and regimental hospitals or subordinate conflicts over therapeutics during this period at face value. While it is undeniable that military medical leaders had strong views about the practice of medicine, it is clear that they were perceived also to be motivated in their impassioned arguments by other, non-medical, considerations. The evidence of the letters written by those men considered below indicates that that perception was most probably correct. Importantly, when considering the practices of the wider military medical community, it would be naive to think that ordinary medical practitioners within the army were unaware of these issues, or that a desire to ingratiate themselves to one or other of these parties did not play some part in the therapeutic choices they made and medical views they expressed.[79]

Disintegration of the Army Medical Board and the Involvement of Parliament

The conflict was moved further outside the medical sphere as the protagonists sought government approbation of their views. At the same time as the undignified pamphlet war was taking place, the government requested an official response from the AMB to the 'Fifth Report'.[80] The ensuing series of letters made clear the importance of patronage to the members of the AMB and, unfortunately for the AMB members, revealed passions so high that concerns were raised about the ability of the AMB to conduct the medical business of the army.

Keate, the AMB member most damaged by the report, was quick to make a detailed response to the government's request. He forwarded eight copies of his *Observations* to the secretary at war for the King and his relevant ministers, and considered, in some detail, the report's proposed changes to the AMD. In that letter, Keate refrained from making the personal attacks characteristic of his other works and concentrated instead on the issues. Keate's argument in defence of general hospitals is thorough and pleads their importance in times of crisis, thus justifying their apparently 'superfluous' existence at other times. Similarly, he rebutted allegations of there being too many medical officers on the grounds of 'the prudence of providing against the worst, rather than for the best'.[81] He gave much attention to the subject of reform of the AMB, not surprisingly arguing against its reconstitution. He stated that any change to the AMB would be misguided and expensive, and deliberately misunderstands the commissioners to have suggested the appointment of a non-medical man to head the AMB. This 'straw man' argument does provide Keate with the excuse to highlight the inability of laymen to understand medical questions (a statement more intriguing in the light of his later appeals to government for adjudication of medical disputes). He also attacked the commissioners for adopting the 'erroneous opinion' that there were 'some peculiarities in army diseases and in their treatment, with which regular physicians were supposed to be unacquainted, and indeed incapable of becoming acquainted'. In this way, Keate is representative of his elite cohort who, paradoxically, asserted specialization in most areas of medical knowledge to protect their own interests, but refused to acknowledge any body of specialized knowledge required for military medicine (presumably because they did not possess any). In keeping with his evidence to the inquiry, he called for a return to the pre-1798 arrangement of the AMB – the joint exercise of powers.

In further requests for submissions from the AMB, the government appeared to be trying to limit the extent of reform, apparently seriously considering merely a return to the pre-1798 arrangement. This proposal was in keeping with the suggestions of Pepys and Keate in their evidence to the commissioners. However, Knight's refusal to co-operate with the request for a joint report from the three members on this question made clear the inability of these AMB members to work together. Despite Secretary at War Sir James Murray-Pulteney's repeated requests for a joint report, and his rejection of individual reports sent to him by the AMB members, Knight refused to comply. Eventually Keate and Pepys were forced to state that they could not get their colleague to sign the propositions they were submitting.[82]

The animosity of Pepys and Keate to Knight and the regimental hospital system found a target following the return of Sir John Moore's shattered army from Corunna in January 1809. The army had been ravaged by typhus on its desperate retreat through the mountains of Spain. Francis Knight's aforementioned closure of the general hospitals in Britain placed those evacuated soldiers in a perilous situation. A bed-crisis threatened and was only averted when McGrigor, in his capacity as inspector of hospitals for the South West district, saved the day and secured places in naval and other institutions for the vast numbers of returned soldiers. However, the near disaster raised questions about Knight's actions and the value of general hospitals to the war effort. In an attempt to capitalize on this circumstance, Pepys and Keate (who had not learned their lesson from the Isle of Wight affair) complained to the government about Knight's handling of the crisis. Once again, their attempts to expose the inadequacies of the regimental model and its advocates backfired.

In April and May that year, the physician general and surgeon general wrote to the secretary at war on matters 'touching the Hospital system on the late service of the Army in Spain and Portugal, and also upon the return of that Army to England'.[83] Knight later stated that those letters alleged his arrangements were defective, encouraging of contagion and responsible for the loss of 1,000 lives.[84] A board of inquiry was established to investigate the matter.[85] The findings of this board exonerated Knight. The Commander in Chief criticized Pepys and Keate who 'should have made themselves more accurately acquainted with the matters contained in their letters and enclosures before they brought them forward for this public investigation'.[86]

The fall-out was serious for the future of the AMB. Knight wrote several outraged letters to government ministers and claimed, point-blank, that the Board could no longer be expected to work together:

> it is impossible for me, either with a view to the advantage of the service, or to the safety of my own character, longer to act in a public capacity with my two Colleagues ...
>
> A new arrangement of the Office, has indeed long been talked of and promised ... I am impelled most seriously to invite the attention of higher authorities to the subject, and to solicit an immediate arrangement that shall completely separate me from two men, whose official conduct has been so offensive to myself as well as to the decorum and discipline of the service.[87]

Predictably, Knight's letters prompted an even longer response from Keate who wrote on 4 August to the secretary at war setting out in extensive detail the part of Knight in the disputes at the AMB. Knight, according to Keate, was 'exclusively chargeable with the blame resulting from this disagreement, as having been the original author and promoter of every thing that has occurred to disturb the harmony of the ... Board'.[88] Keate gave remarkable evidence of bullying tactics and tantrums indulged in by Knight. He asserted that Knight's motivation in all this, particularly in his attempts to encroach on Keate's areas of responsibility, was the cultivation of as much patronage as possible. Keate's criticism was not that Knight was seeking patronage, but that he was seeking more than his fair share. Keate pointed to the closure of general hospitals and Knight's preference for the regimental system in this context, asserting that Knight's preference derived from his ability to exercise and develop patronage in the latter system but not the former. Discussing Knight's creation of the senior position of 'Deputy Inspector' (for which physicians were ineligible) Keate stated:

> in this mode Mr Knight has produced a mischievous division in the Medical Department of the Army, rendering the Physicians on the one hand highly discontented with what they consider as unjust and oppressive treatment, and on the other hand,

gratifying and attaching immediately to himself those whose interests have been promoted by that treatment, and thus constituting himself the head of a party, by which
I have been aggrieved.

He also alleged that Knight engineered the presentation of evidence to the
Commissioners of Military Enquiry intended to:

[disgrace] in the public estimation both General Hospitals and Army Physicians
(which, being under the direction of the Physician General and myself, he desired to
suppress or discard) that those obliging witnesses must have expected at least to recommend themselves strongly to Mr. Knight, by what they did on that occasion; and
such an expectation appears to have been singularly well founded, since Mr. Knight
has continued to be their firm friend and protector.

Keate ends his letter with the ultimatum: either he goes, or we go.

This remarkable series of letters caused significant unease about the AMB
among senior ministers, the secretary at war and commander-in-chief caution-
ing 'the members of the AMB from permitting any difference of opinion among
themselves interfering in the slightest degree with the performance of their duty'.[89]

However, Knight's agitations did not cease and the very day after receiving
this warning he wrote to the adjutant general requesting that the report of the
Board of General Officers be published as a General Order, 'in justice to my
official character, so grievously and insidiously traduced by my Colleagues'.[90] The
following day he wrote to the deputy secretary at war that he hoped he would
not be required to 'act in a Board with the Physician General, and Surgeon General, in which capacity I have no scruple in saying my services can be of no avail,
and I owe it to the public as well as to myself to declare that I cannot act'.[91]
Knight appears to have been gambling that in a restructure of the AMD, he
would be given sole control.

The inability of the AMB to function and the unwillingness of the members
to remedy the breach thus became abundantly clear to senior ministers and they
began to canvas new possible arrangements for the AMD.[92] On 15 August 1809,
the deputy secretary at war communicated to the AMB:

The Secretary at War, in communicating the sentiments of the Commander in Chief,
and his own opinion ... directs me to express his deep regret at the discordance which
exists among the principal officers of the Army Medical Board, especially at a time
when the exigencies of the Service require the most cordial co-operation.

    As it would appear, however, that notwithstanding the caution which was com-
municated on this head in my letter of the 5th of this month, the Inspector General of
Army Hospitals still declines to act with his Colleagues as a Board ... Lord Granville
Levenson Gower, with the concurrence of the Commander in Chief approves of the
arrangement for the care of the sick and wounded expected from the Army under the
command of the Earl of Chatham being carried on by the Surgeon General.[93]

This was the situation of the AMB as the crisis at Walcheren manifested, Knight refused to work with his colleagues and Keate's responsibilities were increased. The principal defence offered by the AMB when questioned about the Walcheren affair was that they had never been informed, nor consulted, about the destination of, nor the possible medical issues that might arise from, Lord Chatham's expedition. It is tempting to posit that the government found the AMB so appallingly ineffective and unprofessional in the months preceding the expedition that such consultation was not even considered. In any event, the actions of the AMB members once the crisis unfolded sealed their fate.

Walcheren was a military disaster, one largely attributable to the incapacity of at times half the force due to disease. It exposed many British doctors to new challenges and was certainly a formative influence on the administrative abilities of McGrigor. However, it is the effect on the AMB which is under consideration in this chapter. The AMB cannot be blamed for the inadequate medical provisioning of the Expedition. Still smarting from the 'Fifth Report', Keate had adopted a 'by-the-book' approach to all his activities and, accordingly, the expedition had the standard medical provisions. However, once the AMB did realize where the expedition had gone they did not sound the alarm with military authorities and claimed, when questioned, that it was not their job to raise matters with government – they were a consultative body only. Once again, this attitude appears to have been taken by Pepys and Keate in response to criticisms levelled at Keate for pre-emptive and 'uneconomical' initiatives he had undertaken in the provisioning of overseas stations. As the crisis worsened, Keate and Pepys do appear to have been quite active in ensuring that the returning troops would be well catered for, and the allegation of 'supineness' levelled at them by several historians cannot be supported.[94]

In late September 1809, the government requested the 'Principal Officer' of the AMB to proceed to Walcheren to investigate the cause and nature of the disease ravaging the troops.[95] This resulted in a flurry of activity within the AMB. Each AMB member devised reasons why he could not possibly go to Walcheren and, in an alliance of convenience, Keate and Knight alleged that the most appropriate member was Pepys.[96] Consequently, the government ordered Pepys to undertake the mission.[97] He responded to this order with a very sensible letter asserting that Knight was the least busy of the AMB members at that time, and recommending the eminent former naval physician Dr Gilbert Blane if Knight refused.[98] This prompted a stern response from the commander-in-chief and the secretary at war stating that the physician general was the most proper officer for the mission and desiring that he go *'immediately'*.[99] This prompted the most extraordinary reply from Pepys:

> *I hereby solemnly declare myself incapable of performing* [this duty], and lament that
> my letter of yesterday was not satisfactory, without being urged to this declaration
> ... I request that Dr. Blane may go as *my substitute* ... whereas if I was able to go, who
> knowing nothing of the investigation of Camp and Contagious Diseases, it would be
> merely pro formâ, and no possible good could arise from it.[100]

This excuse was accepted by the commander-in-chief who instead sent a delegation comprising Sir Gilbert Blane, William Lempriere (also recommended by Pepys) and Robert Jackson's associate, Dr Borland. It must have been particularly galling for Pepys to read the following communication from the government:

> as Inspector Borland has, in the most handsome and zealous manner, offered his ser-
> vices upon this occasion ... express to Doctor Borland that the Commander in Chief
> and the Secretary at War entertain a proper sense of the zeal manifested by him on so
> important a point for the Service.[101]

Knight also made a very 'gallant' offer to go upon hearing of the physician general's refusal.[102] However, it is likely that he was already aware that his services would not be required and his offer merely another of his calculating, self-serving attempts to ingratiate himself with those in power.

The old school/new school politics was evident within the delegation that did go to Walcheren, demonstrating that the conflict did permeate beyond the AMB. Blane left for Walcheren without his two colleagues and sent his own report to the government.[103] This prompted an exasperated response requesting Blane to submit a report in conjunction with Drs Borland and Lempriere.[104]

On this mission, Blane was in constant contact with his establishment colleague Pepys, and in his letters was quick to praise Lempriere for his assistance and 'liberality of mind' but was pointedly silent about Borland.[105] McGrigor, an ally of Knight, had been dispatched to Walcheren to superintend the care and evacuation of the sick. Knight entered into a hostile correspondence with Keate regarding the exercise of McGrigor's duties, and again both insisted on drawing ministers into their quarrel.[106]

McGrigor was later to refer to Pepys' refusal to go to Walcheren as an 'evil hour' and remarked that the actions of the AMB 'excited at the time not only ridicule and contempt, but great indignation was expressed thereat in Parliament'.[107] It has been demonstrated that the reform of the AMB had been under consideration since the 'Fifth Report'. On 25 November 1809, an order was finally given by the commander-in-chief to form a board of officers to 'take into consideration the present state of the medical Department of the Army; and to submit such arrangements as may in their opinion be well adapted for its future government'.[108] Significantly, the board of five officers who would determine the future shape of the AMD did not comprise any medical men. Pepys and Keate continued to write to government ministers, stressing the superiority of general hospitals and 'properly' educated medical officers,[109] but it was to no avail and on 18 December, the Board of General Officers recommended the new AMB, dominated by a director general and assisted by principal inspectors of hospitals.

Predictably, the reactions of the old AMB were less than dignified, Pepys was quick to denigrate the qualifications of Weir, 'a surgeon from Jamaica' for the directorship, and both he and Keate wrote plaintive letters to the secretary at war about their retirement entitlements.[110] The issue which had dominated the Board's time in office was addressed by Pepys in an extraordinary letter to the secretary at war. In it he explicitly stated that it had been his intention while in office to improve the quality of army medical care by populating the physicians' posts with graduates of Cambridge, Oxford and Dublin universities. Furthermore he criticized competence of the AMB who had made the decision and its plan to commit the care of the army to regimental surgeons:

> The Board about to be established under your Lordship's sanction propose to have the care of the Army committed entirely to Regimental Surgeons. Whether your Lordship was of opinion, that previous Academical Education is necessary or advisable before the Study of Medicine in the Medical Schools, either here or at Edinburgh, I wished to know when I had the honour of waiting on your lordship lately, but as I found you declined to enter on the subject, I thought it my duty ... to trouble your Lordship with this, that it might hereafter be known that I had expressed my opinion in writing on this important subject. A Board of General Officers determining on the Medical Arrangements of the Army, is not more incompetent than a College of Physicians to decide on the attack of a fortress. As the Commander in Chief disavows the intended change, as originating with Him, your Lordship will see the propriety of my addressing you, before it is too late, to request that the abolition of regularly educated Physicians from the Army may be well considered by your Lordship and also ... Mr Keate's printed observations, where your Lordship will see the consequence when surgeons called Physicians, but not really so, act as Physicians.[111]

These actions by the AMB during possibly the worst medical crisis yet encountered by the British forces during the Wars, came under close scrutiny during the Walcheren inquiry and the questions directed to the participants reveal the interest government was beginning to take in medical questions and the running of the AMD. In particular, clear concerns were expressed about the inability of the service to attract hospital mates[112] and ongoing invalidism of returned troops representing a significant loss to the British army.[113] Questions directed to John Webb, the deputy inspector of hospitals at Walcheren, pointedly exhibited government interest in the actions taken by doctors to prevent and control the spread of disease.[114] Both in the inquiry and in Parliament, the focus of the opposition was to show that if different military decisions had been taken, and the army pushed forward to Antwerp, disease would not have struck and the operation would have been more likely to succeed. Nevertheless, it is clear that Parliament was beginning to take a strong interest in the therapeutic choices made by medical officers, and to question their appropriateness in light of the effects disease could exact on the strength of Britain's fighting forces. The interest of politicians in the medical services provided for soldiers appears to also have been prompted by the public outcry about the matter after the calamity at Walcheren became widely known.[115]

Conclusion

A history of the AMB leading up to the crisis at Walcheren demonstrates that while, in the public eye, Walcheren may have caused the breaking up of the AMB, it was really the tail end of a story extending back over the previous ten years. By the time the AMB exhibited its ineffectiveness at Walcheren, the government was already taking steps to reconstitute it. Regardless, the 'breaking' of the Board is not the most important consequence of this ten-year period for the history of military medicine. The tenure of the Board was during a period of massive influx into the AMD from non-elite institutions and apprentice backgrounds. New recruits gained experience overseas and 'on-the-field'; many were seeking a better life and status. In part, this explosion of medical officers explains the movement led by men like Jackson for the recognition of regimental hospitals and regimental experience. As McGrigor later admitted, the furiousness of the debate was curious as both regimental and general hospitals were needed during the war. This influx of practitioners also explains the forming of alliances and the creation of an alternate patronage network to the 'old school' of Pepys.

Crucially, the majority of these debates centred on whether military medicine required specialized knowledge and training. The military medicine that emerged during these wars challenged the old model both intellectually and in the crucial arenas of status, money and authority. The fracturing of medical authority into two distinct camps and the notoriousness of the dispute might have contributed to therapeutic choices made by young doctors; choices that would have set them on intellectual pathways for the duration of their careers, extending in many cases long after the Wars had finished. These political, status-linked matters must be borne in mind and provide an important backdrop to the changes and debates in medicine that will be considered in the following chapters over the period of the Wars and into the first half of the nineteenth century.

3 EGYPT, OPHTHALMIA AND PLAGUE

Previous chapters have claimed that the challenges of military medical practice in foreign climates were significant factors in the production of the belief that military medicine was specialized and distinct from civilian practice. This chapter will investigate that process through a detailed examination of the Egyptian campaign and its consequences in Britain.

The Egyptian campaign began in July 1798 when Napoleon and his 'Army of the Orient' arrived there with the intention of conquering the region and then making for British possessions in India.[1] Although initially successful, a series of defeats in 1799 prevented the French army from achieving its goal. Unable to return to France after Nelson famously destroyed the French fleet at Abukir Bay, the army was abandoned by Napoleon who slipped back to Paris in August that year. Under General Kleber and (after Kleber's assassination) General Menou, the French army remained in Egypt for another two years. In 1801, the British sent Lt General Sir Ralph Abercrombie with 16,000 men to remove the threat presented to India by the remaining French troops in Egypt. Additional British and Indian troops were sent from India. After a series of engagements, during which Abercrombie was killed and Major General Hutchinson took charge of the British forces, the French surrendered and towards the end of 1801 both armies began their journeys home.[2]

This campaign has been described by some historians as not only geographically, but also militarily, peripheral to the Wars.[3] Whatever the merits of this general assessment, it could not be less appropriate to the development of British military medicine. In Egypt, both armies were afflicted with severe and persistent dysentery and diarrhoea. Medical practitioners were confronted by a harsh and unfamiliar climate and diseases of which they had almost no medical knowledge and certainly no experience, such as the plague and Egyptian ophthalmia. This latter disease was carried by armies back to their home countries and after the campaign it ran rampant in British military garrisons and infiltrated the British civilian population. It is largely this aspect of the Egyptian campaign which has attracted the interest of medical historians, who have identified the epidemic as the genesis of specialist ophthalmic hospitals and the emergence of specialist ophthalmologists.[4]

Other medical aspects of the campaign have received less attention from historians. Cantlie and Kempthorne provide detailed narratives of the movements of the armies, and accounts of the diseases encountered and the casualties suffered, but do not venture far on issues such as the implications of the campaign for the development of British army medicine.[5] The biographers of prominent physicians who served on the campaign also go into some detail about the problems, privations and medical victories of those men in Egypt; however, their accounts are largely just replications of those physicians' autobiographies.[6]

Encounters with ophthalmia and other diseases during the British armies' time in Egypt influenced the practice of medicine in later campaigns and the development of medical thought. Arguably, the campaign was formative for McGrigor who was, at this time, in charge of the medical services for the Indian army. It is very likely his experiences in Egypt helped to shape not only his talent for military medical administration, but also influenced his approach to therapeutics and medical reasoning. His records, and the writings of other practitioners on the campaign, also how army doctors approached the investigation of 'new' diseases, giving some insight into the investigative processes and medical philosophies of these men.

These processes and philosophies were important building blocks in the construction of army medical officers' argued positions in later debates over their medical superiority to civilian practitioners. These aspects of the campaign will be considered in the first half of this chapter. More attention is given in this section to the treatments used by practitioners than elsewhere. It is intended that this will demonstrate the diversity and independence of practice amongst practitioners in the British army early in the 1800s, and also to help identify how practitioners were influenced by each other and by the French. In an era when British practitioners could not travel to Paris to study medicine, or collaborate with French colleagues, the interaction between the two professional groups in Egypt is significant. The emergence of hospital medicine in France has been closely linked to developments in French military medicine during this period.

The spread of Egyptian ophthalmia throughout the British army when it returned to Britain will be examined in the second half of the chapter. However, instead of focusing on the development of ophthalmology as a specialization (which has already been extensively researched) it will consider how military medical officers applied the experience they had gained in Egypt to practice in Britain. It will show how a growing identification of the disease with filth and contagion superseded climatic theories of disease which had previously been favoured. Finally, the attempts of senior army medical officers to control and standardize the treatment of the disease will be investigated.

The story of the Egyptian ophthalmia is taken up again in Chapter 6 which considers a contest over the 'territory' of ophthalmia between the military medical establishment and civilian doctors immediately after the Wars.

French Medical Practitioners in Egypt

The French army arrived in Egypt well in advance of the British. It endured long marches through the deserts, deprivation and thirst, sieges and battles. It did not take long for the routine army diseases, dysentery and diarrhoea, to appear. In 1798, practitioners began to report that a distinctly unfamiliar disease, ophthalmia, was attacking many soldiers and, more alarmingly, plague was also reported. French medical practitioners had been charged by Napoleon not only with the medical care of the army but, like the commissioners of Arts and Sciences accompanying the expedition, also with the collection of data on Egypt and its people. Accordingly, they gathered and published a great deal of information about the diseases of Egypt and their attempts to treat soldiers and locals suffering from them. These works, along with Prosper Alpinus's sixteenth-century text *De Medicina Egyptiorum*,[7] became important references for British army practitioners who looked in desperation for authority on the 'new diseases', plague and ophthalmia, when they spread amongst the British with alarming ferocity.

It was reported by the French that their medical reports and directives were found and used by the British on taking over French hospitals.[8] Sir Sydney Smith collected the French works on ophthalmia and sent them to Dr Gilbert Blane, requesting that he translate and send them back to Egypt for the benefit of the army.[9] There is also evidence that the British and French practitioners discussed the treatment of patients in Egypt.[10] French authority is often cited by British practitioners who published accounts of the Egyptian ophthalmia after the campaign, and some British officers appear to have been strongly influenced by French theories on the diseases of Egypt.[11] This evidence strongly suggests that, in this theatre at least, French medicine had a profound influence on British practice. French publications were also important sources used by British physicians treating ophthalmia in the decades after the campaign. Accordingly, it is important to consider the works of the French before moving on to the British experience in Egypt.

French medicine during this period has been considered by historians to have been strongly influenced by a new 'hospital medicine', grounded in observation and hospital training.[12] Centred on the new Paris hospital, and the teachings of Pinel and Bichat, this medical philosophy was strongly supported in military hospitals, particularly in Montpellier where many of the French practitioners on this expedition had worked.[13] This new medicine is thought to have focused less on medicines and drugs (particularly strong substances) and more on supporting the body's own response (or more severely, simply on dissecting the body once it had expired). This assessment is borne out in part by French practice in Egypt, but tempered in the case of ophthalmia by evidence of the use of various drugs such as sulpher, mercury, aluminium and opiates. In addition, the French were instructed to take an interest in the traditional cures for disease used by local practitioners in Egypt.[14] They did so, experimented with them and incorporated some local methods into their practice.

The physician-in-chief of the French army was Renée Desgenettes, and under him was the surgeon-in-chief, August Larrey. Both products of the new hospital medicine, Desgenettes and Larrey demonstrated a commitment to observation and dissection over theory and to the promotion of health through hygiene. Desgenettes, in particular, expressed his adherence to these principles and encouraged his doctors to follow them. He was assiduous in promoting the collection of topographical, ethnographical and anecdotal information about Egypt and the dissemination of the reports that came in to his medical corps.[15] The opinions and reports of those French practitioners while in Egypt will now be examined, first considering the plague and then ophthalmia.

The French reaction to the plague recorded by Larrey in his *Memoirs of Military Surgery* is important to the history of anticontagionism.[16] Larrey first reported an occurrence of the plague just prior to the undertaking of the march through Syria. He stated that he 'learned from Alexandria, Damietta, and Mansouri, that a pestilential fever attended with carbuncles, and buboes in the groin and axilla, had appeared in these cities and had proved very fatal'.[17] The same symptoms affected a soldier who entered his hospital in Cairo, and Larrey responded by burning the man's effects and the furniture of his bed, ventilating and fumigating his room. He told only Desgenettes of his conviction that the soldier had died from the 'legitimate plague'. He took care not to name the disease 'plague' in the circular to his surgeons, directing them to 'attend with particular care to individuals attacked by this disease, always taking precautions to prevent contagion'.[18] Such cases continued to present themselves during the march through Syria, and at Jaffa the disease reached worrying proportions. Richardson states that Bonaparte instructed that: 'the men had to believe they were suffering from ... a well recognized but non-contagious disease: "fever of the buboes", a disease that in some strange way affected those who lacked courage or whose spirit was weak'.[19]

Larrey appears to have initially concurred with the General's views and in his circular to the surgeons of the army from St Jean d'Acre on 22 March 1799, he referred to it only as 'the reigning disease' and instructed the surgeons:

> This disease, when it has arrived to a certain stage, is contagious; therefore it is necessary to take proper precautions for guarding against it; it is also necessary to make the

soldiers, whose health is committed to your care, observe these precautions, without informing them of the motives.[20]

Larrey later recorded his regret for promoting this policy of disinformation, which resulted in the soldiers not hesitating 'to use the effects of their dead companions', thereby catching the plague. Larrey supported his position by stating that once the soliders were told 'the character of this disease ... they used the precautions pointed out for their preservation'.[21]

In this light, the dominant position taken amongst French medical practitioners in Egypt (i.e. that the plague was not contagious) takes on a different character. Two highly memorable anticontagionist public relations exercises on the campaign: Napoleon's visit to the plague hospital at Cairo;[22] and the 'plague innoculation' performed in front of the troops by Desgenettes on himself, are perhaps more indicative of a militarily-inspired policy than actual medical philosophy.[23] Many anticontagionists of the period drew on the actions of Desgenettes to support their position; however, Desgenettes said himself that he did, in fact, believe the plague to be contagious in certain conditions, 'La peste est évidement contagieuse; mais les conditions de la transmission de cette contagion ne sont pas plus exactement connues que sa nature spécifique'.[24] Contagionists often argued that he only performed the inoculation as a stunt, and was careful to wash the 'pricked' area thoroughly once out of sight of the troops. Desgenettes did state that he performed the inoculation, 'pour rassurer les imaginations et le courage ébranlé de l'armée'.[25] The politicization/militarization of the contagion issue thus revealed, must force the historian to reconsider the anticontagionist positions of Desgenettes and other famous anticontagionst practitioners of this army, such as Assalini.[26] Certainly, the preventative measures imposed on the local population by the French, such as exposing clothing to the sun for long periods and the fumigation of houses, indicate that the possibility of contagion was seriously entertained by even those practitioners who publicly denounced it.[27]

To investigate the disease Larrey 'examined the intestines of the dead, for the causes and effects of the Plague', but without success.[28] He concluded that it was definitely contagious but only in specific circumstances. His writings on the plague while in Egypt advocated the use of vomits and light bleeding in the early stages of the disease, and stressed the importance of keeping the bowels free. He suggested the use of local bitters in large doses in the second stage of the disease combined with suitable topical applications designed to 'assist nature' to excite the suppuration of the buboes. If the patient suffered instead from carbuncles he recommended their scarification and an application of concentrated acid. The strength of the patient was to be supported by bitters and coffee.[29] He thought the plague could be prevented by segregating the infected and by cleanliness. Frequent washing with cold water and vinegar, clean clothes and regimen were his primary recommendations. Above all he insisted that the soldiers be convinced not to sleep in the holes which they dug in the sand. In common with many French practitioners in Egypt, who strongly associated its climate and topography with disease, he felt that the south wind, or 'Khampsin', was an important causative factor in the disease.[30]

Dr Antonio Savaresi, based in Damietta, observed that the 'epidemic fever' (plague) was caused by the winds of the south, rain, humidity, and the fog. His enquiries of the local inhabitants suggested that the best preservative was to wash the head frequently with cold water.[31] Larrey and most other practitioners gave some consideration to the cures employed by the native peoples and tried to use local herbs and fruits in their cures. Both Assalini and Desgenettes experimented with 'frictions of oil'.[32] Assalini recommended gentle evacuations, some bloodletting only of strong men, and the excitement of perspiration and sweating with an almond emulsion mixed with laudanum.[33] Assalini believed that the most effective treatment of epidemic diseases was the banishment of fear, casting doubt once again on the motive behind his commitment to the non-contagiousness of the plague.[34]

The French works on plague were dismissed by some British practitioners, who were 'disappointed to find that so little light has been thrown on plague by the result of the French practitioners in Egypt'.[35] However, the British did learn from the French about what did not work, native cures, methods of prevention and, as already noted, the French experience was very influential to post-campaign debates on contagion. The French writings on ophthalmia were better received by the British.

The accounts of ophthalmia by French practitioners in Egypt state that from the beginning of 1798 to the end of 1799, over two thirds of their army suffered from this disease, which could lead to blindness. Their descriptions of the disease, which are similar to those given by British practitioners, represent it as being very painful, having a sudden onset and often causing extreme inflammation and swelling in parts of the eye, nasty suppurations and possible rupture of the cornea.[36] Not surprisingly, significant amounts were written regarding its cause and treatment.

The only author that the French could consult regarding the ophthalmia was Prosper Alpinus. He had identified ophthalmia as a disease endemic to the region caused by the 'poussière nitreuse qui picote et enflame continuellement les yeux des habitants'.[37] He also believed that the strong sun, burning winds and climate of Egypt resulted in eye fatigue, making the eyes susceptible to the ophthalmia. The French incorporated these ideas into their theories, Savaresi in particular adopting a chemical approach to the analysis of the atmosphere (although contradicting Alpinus's findings). However, most French practitioners identified suppressed perspiration as the principle causative factor. This theory was pursued by practitioners who, like Larrey, believed that ophthalmia was linked to the local dysentery, and could be caused by its sudden suppression.

Savaresi's work on the Egyptian ophthalmia is often cited in later British works, and in doctoral theses of the period. His chemical analysis led him to conclude that clay and chalk combined with carbonic acid and lime in the atmosphere of Egypt caused the disease. He arrived at this conclusion by testing that concoction on the eyes of some unfortunate local dogs.[38] In his work he divided the disease into sthenic and asthenic types and began the treatment of each with a purge, 'une once de sulfate de magnésie' followed by bleeding at the temple.[39] Interestingly, the division of the disease into sthenic and asthenic types strongly reflects the medical philosophy of John Brown known as 'Brunonianism'. Brown had been a student of Cullen at Edinburgh in the late 1700s, but rejected Cullen's complex nosology and instead asserted that all disease was the result of changes in the degree of a person's 'excitement'. Accordingly, Brown advocated the use of stimulants to cure disease. Comments by McGrigor discussed later in this chapter suggest that the Brunonian system was advocated by a small but significant number of British regimental surgeons during this campaign, and (to a lesser extent) it is also apparent later in the Wars. This may reflect the popularity of the system among what Rosner terms a 'vocal minority' of students at Edinburgh in the 1780s where many regimental surgeons would have trained. The system's simplicity may also have appealed to military surgeons for its ease of application in the difficult circumstances on campaign. If the bleeding did not have an effect within an hour he recommended a moderate regime and the use of calming collyria. In the second type he recommended collyria of suplhate of zinc in vinegar and l'eau de vie.[40]

Citizen Bruant, a young surgeon who died of the plague in Egypt, also wrote an influential paper on the ophthalmia. In it, he identified Alpinus's scorching nitrous dust and the united fatiguing actions of heat and light on the eyes as the culprits in the majority of cases. He also identified a second, less common, type of ophthalmia linked with dysentery, which was caused by 'acrid bilious sordes in the primae viae'. A third type attacked persons of a delicate habit. He believed that it was impossible to prevent the disease as its causes were everywhere in the environment, so instead favoured a programme to moderate their effects. Because of its simplicity and ease of incorporation into a soldier's routine, he especially advocated frequent washing of the eyes with cold water. In keeping with the 'new hospital medicine', Bruant claimed that the condition often resolved itself 'without having recourse to art and one may say, with truth, that nothing so much stands in the way of a cure, as a multiplicity of remedies, especially external applications'. However, he did argue that it was important to facilitate the body's own response, by keeping the bowels open with a decoction of tamarinds and other laxative ptisans. He thought that bleeding from the arm could be of use, but that it was counter-indicated by the weakened state of the soldiers. In difficult cases he recommended topical bleeding as practised by the locals. In general his only treatment was to remove the eye from all irritating stimuli, especially light. Once the inflammation abated he used resolvent collyria, gradually rendered stronger to complete the cure.[41]

Assalini considered the ophthalmia 'a true defluxion of humors', and while he thought the bright lights, dust and sand of Egypt were detrimental to the eye, he argued that the primary cause of the disease, just as in the case of dysentery, was suppressed perspiration. He records treating 2,000 patients with the disease and only losing one to blindness. He believed that bleeding was a waste of time, but because all the patients wanted it, he substituted general bleeding with leeches, scarifications, blisters and finally setons. In a simple ophthalmia he used a weak solution of verdigrisse and prohibited the washing of the eyes, whilst also keeping them out of the light. In a complicated ophthalmia he believed the stomach could become affected and so it was necessary to use soporifics and bloodletting. He investigated the cures used by Egyptians, and while dismissing many of them as being ineffective and responsible for the large numbers of blind in the country, did agree that emollients, cataplasms and water were harmful in this disease. Most strongly, he recommended a collyrium of verdigrisse, the wearing of green spectacles and never sleeping in the open air as preventative measures.[42]

Finding that there were many different opinions within the army as to the cause and treatment of the ophthalmia, Larrey thought it 'proper to publish a memoir ... in order to establish a proper mode of treatment'. It is this memoir that he alleged was found and used by the British when they took over the hospital at Rosetta. In it he stated that the cause of the ophthalmia was the effect of suppressed perspiration on eyes already weakened by the vivid rays of the sun in Egypt. Similarly he believed that the sudden suppression of diarrhoea or gonorrhoea could have the same effect. Although he believed that serous ophthalmia could 'terminate by means of perspiration, superabundance of tears, and especially by diarrhoea',[43] he stated that inflammatory ophthalmia 'seldom terminates well, without the assistance of art'.[44] For inflammatory ophthalmia, Larrey recommended bloodletting in the veins of the neck, arm or foot and then the application of leeches to the temples as near to the eye as possible. He also added a pediluvium to these prescriptions and the 'steam of a decoction of emollient and anodyne substances should be directed on the eye ... it should be washed with a strong decoction of flaxseed, poppy, and oriental safron [*sic*]'.[45] Stronger substances used by Larrey included sulphate of alumen and camphor. He also concurred that it was important to keep the patient out of the light. As the condition improved he advocated the use of stronger collyria adding acetate of lead or a weak solution of oxygenated muriate or mercury or sulphate of copper to the mix. In the most obstinate cases he resorted to surgery to reduce the swollen eyelids and conjunctiva. In the case of ophthalmia resulting from the suppression of gonorrhoea he recommended the inoculation anew with matter of gonorrhoea, and in cases resulting from gastric affection vomits, purges and bitter drinks.[46]

Desgenettes took the findings of many doctors regarding the dangers of suppressed perspiration very seriously. He issued orders emphasizing the importance of keeping covered at night, and not sleeping without clothes. In his opinion, those who did not suffered from derangements in perspiration which could produce many sicknesses, including ophthalmia, diahorrea and dysentery.[47] The theory of suppressed perspiration provided an overriding explanation of the Egyptian diseases – plague, ophthalmia and dysentery – and made strong links between them. It drew strongly on the Egyptian environment of sudden temperature changes and moist dews at night. It seems to have been the most widely held theory by the French doctors, and was picked up by the British.

The influence of the French theories on the Egyptian diseases can be seen most clearly in the various treatments tried by the British for ophthalmia. As seen above, some British physicians acknowledged the French in their publications; others like McGrigor rarely did. However, that lack of acknowledgment does not mean that the observations of French physicians, which we know were communicated to them, were not considered as they struggled to deal with the Egyptian diseases. In the case of plague, the British benefited from reading the research carried out by the French, but they took a significantly more interventionist approach to the cure of the disease. The hospitals established by the French in Egyptian towns and the practices they had enforced among the local populations were also useful to the British. Additionally, the French experience in Egypt provided British practitioners who investigated these diseases after the Wars with important points of reference.

James McGrigor and the Plague in Egypt

As noted above, the British sent two armies to Egypt. The first, under Abercrombie landed at Aboukir Bay on 8 March 1801, the other led by General Baird journeyed from India to Cosseir on the Red Sea, and then had to march across the 120 miles of desert from Cossier to the Nile. In an astonishing feat of organization, the army travelling by night achieved this end with only one casualty. Not long after landing in Egypt, over 25 per cent of the first British force was in hospital, struck down with diarrhoea, dysentery and fever. Some units had nearly 40 per cent of men off duty. Hospitals were crowded with over 3,000 cases and there were 1,182 in the hospital ships. The more severe cases were shipped to Malta, Gibraltar and England. To defeat the French at Cairo, the army advanced up the Nile Valley in May. A covering force of 6,000 men was left to contain the French isolated in Alexandria and troops were pushed on to occupy Rosetta. On the slow and hot march up the Nile, plague and ophthalmia began to affect the troops.[48]

The principal medical officer of Abercrombie's force was initially Dr James Franck,[49] who was later replaced by Dr Thomas Young. The chief medical officer of Baird's force was supposed to be Dr Shapter, who was sent out from England with a medical staff and equipment, but his superintendence was suspended in favour of McGrigor until the army reached Lower Egypt. Franck and Shapter both continued to serve with their armies, despite their demotions. Both seem to have been well respected gentlemen of ability, but they lacked military experience and, importantly, did not have relationships of influence with Abercrombie or Baird. Both were replaced at the behest of these men. Abercrombie used his influence to have Franck replaced by Young, who had served with Abercrombie in the West Indies and at the Helder. Young was not popular with the AMB; he had made a practice of defying its instructions, especially in the promotion of his own men, but he was clearly popular with Abercrombie who was of a similar mind.

McGrigor considered the relationship between the commander of a force, and its chief medical officer was important to the maintenance of soldiers' health. It is not unlikely that McGrigor, and others like Young, were also strongly aware of the importance of these relationships to their careers. McGrigor would probably have argued that the two were interlinked, success in each area being mutually reinforcing. As we have seen, his attitude to military health gave much importance to, and incorporated, military culture. As will be demonstrated below, McGrigor attributed much disease within armies to the effects of the environments in which they served. In consequence, he reasoned that the prevention of disease was strongly associated with the regulation of a soldier's personal environment, his hygiene and routine. The soldier's personal environment was, he believed, within the control of his commander: 'The prevention of disease is usually the province, and is mostly in the power, of the military officer; the cure lies with the medical'.[50] McGrigor's emphasis on preventative medicine is explained by his assessment of available cures: 'everything can be done in the prevention of disease; but, unfortunately, very little in the treatment when it supervenes'.[51] Accordingly, McGrigor's energies were concentrated on the acquisition of authority to enforce preventative measures. He sought physical authority to control the men by courting the support of military leaders for his proposals. He also pursued intellectual authority among his colleagues to support the medical theories on which his preventative measures were based. As will be seen in Chapter 5, McGrigor had extraordinarily good relationships with his military commanders throughout his career. It may be that his approach to the treatment of disease began with the cultivation of those relationships. His understanding of the environmental causes of disease and the importance of personal environmental solutions, possibly led him to the conclusion that it was paramount to mould the political environment in which he worked.

McGrigor's influence on military medicine during and after the Wars was profound. In particular, the methods he adopted to help him acquire medical authority had a significant effect on the way military medical knowledge was disseminated as well as the standardization of treatments. Accordingly, it is important to understand his approach to the investigation and treatment of disease. One of the first opportunities he had to direct the operations of a large number of medical officers was on the Egyptian campaign, and it was also here that he really began to implement some of what were to become his characteristic administrative innovations.

McGrigor wrote two accounts of his experiences in Egypt. The first, a report to the Bombay Medical Board, was reproduced in the *Edinburgh Medical and Surgical Journal*.[52] The second, *Medical Sketches of the Expedition from Egypt to India*, has been described by Blanco as 'a landmark in military medicine ... a comprehensive medical history of a significant campaign in an exotic environment [which] also provided military officers with practical lessons in Army Hygiene'.[53] McGrigor's works set out not only his views on the origin and nature of the diseases encountered by the British medical corps, but also how he gathered and distributed information and how he went about investigating 'some of the diseases of Egypt [which were] new to every one of the medical gentlemen'.[54]

The clearest description of McGrigor's investigative process does not relate to any of the Egyptian diseases, but rather to one his regiment, the Connaught Rangers, suffered in India and on the voyage to Egypt – the guinea worm or dracunculus.[55] This worm caused considerable pain and difficulty for the men who were attacked by it. The first sign of the worm was an itching followed by a blister (usually on the leg) after which the end of the worm would poke out of the affected limb. McGrigor admits that on first encountering it he was 'very embarrassed' that he knew so little of it. However, he did believe that it was contagious, and accordingly separated the sick from the sound, increased cleanliness and ventilation on the ship, and washed the decks with boiling water and nitrous fumigants. He required everyone to wash their hands and feet daily and take three baths per week. He states that by following this regime incidents of the disease decreased. To treat those who were affected he consulted his books looking 'in vain for an account of this loathsome and painful disease [finding] mention merely of its name in antiquity, and that the only treatment was to pull it out daily'.[56] He tried to copy the 'Hindoo doctors' in drawing the worm from the leg in two sections, cutting it at its middle. He made experiments on the worm, trying leeches, astringents, sedative lotions and electricity, none of which had much effect. He also tried a mercurial ointment that he believed to be quite good.[57] These experiments were also recorded by Ninian Bruce, another surgeon with the Connaught Rangers, who mentions using aloe leaves, soap-berries and cut up onions on the wound but who questioned the efficacy of mercury in killing the worm.[58]

McGrigor used these same processes – first enforcing segregation and hygienic practices at the onset of any disease, consulting written authorities and then the collection and collation of information through experiment and observation of local practices – in his approach to plague and ophthalmia in Egypt.

Many doctors subsequently published works on the ophthalmia and dysentery of Egypt, but McGrigor is almost the only British practitioner to have written about the plague during the Egyptian campaign. Fortunately, in his work, McGrigor recorded the practices of other practitioners serving with him.

The plague first came to McGrigor's attention in Egypt when the hospital cook and another hospital worker at Rosetta became unwell in September 1801.[59] Prepared for this eventuality, McGrigor had with him Dr Russell's history of the plague, which he often consulted.[60] In his book, Russell strongly argued that the plague was contagious (though affected by climate). McGrigor's environment-controlling, hygienic line of defence swung into action, backed by regulations issued by General Baird.[61] McGrigor quickly moved the men to an extremity of the town. A room was set aside to observe suspect cases within the Rangers and any cases found were immediately sent to the pest-house on the edge of town, the building was cleaned with a nitrous fumigation, and after everyone's clothes had been washed, hair cut and body bathed they were moved to a new building. Similar measures were used throughout the campaign whenever a suspected case of plague was identified.

Unfortunately, his efforts did not completely succeed in stopping the spread of the plague, and by April the following year it was present not only in Rosetta but had travelled as far 'as Aboukir on the one side, and ... Rahamania on the other side of Alexandria; and we had information that most of the intermediate stages, betwixt us and these two places, were infected'.[62] Accordingly, McGrigor established quarantines on people travelling between cities.

Once this line of defence had been established McGrigor turned his mind to the much more difficult task of investigating and finding a cure for the disease. In addition to consulting written authorities on the plague, he directed investigations into the nature of the plague, the conduct of dissections on plague victims and the trial of different cures.[63] His method was explicitly collaborative. He collected the research of other medical practitioners in Egypt from their reports and letters, particularly those working in the pest establishments, and had them sewn together so that any other medical gentlemen could 'come and peruse them'. By this method, he intended that the disease would become a subject of discussion and that drawing on that discussion he could then pose questions for investigation to the men working in the pest houses.[64] His confidence in this method is borne out in his final work on the subject:

> The Sketches which I mean to give of the plague, I draw principally from the reports made to me by the surgeons of the army, and from a pretty voluminous correspondence with the gentlemen whose names have already been mentioned. From my own experience I hardly can venture to speak: it was very limited. Though I saw a great many cases, in the first stage of the disease, the number of cases which I treated throughout was very small; they were the cases which first appeared in the army, and my success in them leaves me little to boast of. The reports and statements of the different gentlemen I have compared together, and endeavoured to reconcile them by what I myself saw of many of the cases.[65]

This belief in the importance of the centralization of information and experience is an important aspect of McGrigor's approach to medicine and the duties of a military practitioner:

> I think it a matter of regret that such journals are not more frequently kept; with a little industry on the part of the profession they might always be so. Had such records been always faithfully kept, many practical points would not, as they now are, be involved in doubt and uncertainty. We should not now be so ignorant of some diseases, of the countries where we have so often made campaigns, or of which we have so long been in the possession. Humble as the labours may seem, and confined as the abilities of an individual may be, were he only faithfully to relate observations made with care, to compare them with those of his contemporaries, and by these to correct the opinions of his predecessors, he would perform no mean service to his art.[66]

Such faith in the revelatory power of collected experience is possibly related to the faith McGrigor put in the power of statistics to reveal truths about disease. He had, earlier in his career, found a fascination with the collection of information and statistics to contribute to the understanding of disease. Blanco argues that this is evidence of McGrigor's 'empirical attitude towards medicine, a sceptical view of traditional systems of the monistic pathology of disease, an emphasis on more accurate clinical observations, and a stress upon autopsies'.[67] However, McGrigor reveals here that his first purpose in the collection of experience was the distribution of that experience; the centralization of knowledge to distil and then disseminate it. There was significant power inherent in his method to control the direction of medical knowledge and he used it quite successfully to promote the therapeutic use of mercury (which he recommended in the treatment of almost any affliction) for the Egyptian diseases.

McGrigor's record also details experiments that did not work, and some that he would have liked to have undertaken, but could not. He believed that cold bathing would have been an effective cure for the plague but never got to test it.[68] The dissections, which McGrigor believed to have rarely been performed on plague victims before, had to be stopped because they made the dissectors unwell.[69]

Some methods of treatment were very unsuccessful, as McGrigor reports it, particularly those based in Brunonianism and anticontagionism. McGrigor seems to have been theoretically opposed to Brunonianism, and especially to the use of bloodletting by the Brunonian, Dr Whyte, stating simply, 'all his patients died'.[70] McGrigor also recorded the failure of stimulants to treat the plague:

> Some gentlemen, attached to the Brunonian system, put the stimulating plan to the test. By Messieurs Adrian and Whyte, patients were for some time kept under the influence of wine and opium; but, this practice was never successful and they deserted it. It was at length the practice of Mr Adrian to unite stimulants and mercurials.[71]

McGrigor's approach was based implicitly on most diseases being contagious.[72] Despite the prevailing belief amongst the British that the plague was definitely contagious, some doctors believed otherwise. The most prominent of these was Dr Daniel Whyte, who prior to the campaign had been a naval surgeon and travelled of his own accord in the region. He served with the Maltese corps and at some point had had the medical charge of about 1,000 of the sailors on the transports.[73]

Whyte turns up in almost every medical account of the expedition. He was one of the 'gentlemen, attached to the Brunonian system' within the medical corps.[74] He had novel treatments for most of the Egyptian diseases; in particular, his approaches to dysentery and ophthalmia were much discussed and emulated by many surgeons on the expedition. According to Henry Dewar he was, 'a man of acuteness, but rather of an eccentric turn', who, despite his apparent influence, was not liked by many of his fellow practitioners in Egypt.[75] Whyte's ironic fate throughout the first half of the nineteenth century was to become one of the most commonly cited examples used to prove that the plague was contagious. Like Desgenettes, Whyte had proposed to prove the non-contagious nature of the plague by inoculating himself with the pus from a buboe. He was cautioned against it by Dr Wittman, but went ahead regardless.[76] Unfortunately for Whyte, on his second or third trial of this process he contracted the plague and died. McGrigor states that Whyte 'fell a martyr to his zeal in the investigation of the history of the plague'.[77]

The results of all this discussion and investigation were, according to McGrigor, threefold. It revealed some new facts about the disease, achieved a generally agreed treatment and demonstrated that plague could be managed, the huge mortality rate in local populations being only the result of 'gross ignorance'.

The generally agreed treatment required first a purge of calomel, then the inducement of ptyalism and perspiration by nitric acid given internally, or bathing patients in citric acid and vinegar. Thirdly, to obviate debility the patient was given bark, wine and opium. McGrigor stated that 'on the whole, in mercury and the nitric acid, we appear to have excellent remedies for the plague: but they must be very early and very liberally exhibited'.[78] However, it was in the prevention and arrest of the plague that McGrigor believed the British had triumphed:

> It is a matter of no little consolation to us, that we know the means, not only of excluding the plague from our own country, but that, when our armies are stationed in the countries where the disease is endemic, we can arrest the progress of the contagion, and with certainty eradicate it.[79]

It is significant that McGrigor attached so much importance to these successes in prevention and of removing the widespread dread that traditionally accompanied plague. In this he exhibited not only his medical but also his military colours. McGrigor was strongly focused on the preservation of fighting troops in tropical climates and, despite admitting only limited success in curing the plague, he believed that the venture had been enormously successful because he had learned to prevent the disease.

Ophthalmia in Egypt

McGrigor displayed the same practical approach to the importance of prevention in his conclusion on ophthalmia:

> By an attention to [Dr Whyte's] mode of prevention, and in the season when the ophthalmia prevails most, making the soldiers wear something over the eyes, I think we should have the prospect of passing a second campaign, or season in Egypt, with less loss from ophthalmia.[80]

The Egyptian ophthalmia 'prevailed very generally' among the British troops almost as soon as they arrived in Egypt.[81] It was 'after the Plague, the most formidable disease in the army, from its general prevalence'. By October that first year McGrigor reported 'the number of cases of ophthalmia and the great degree of violence in which this disease was now seen, were really alarming'.[82] He stated that the medical men of the British army followed very different treatments for ophthalmia, and in keeping with his approach to the plague, he recorded many of those treatments in his discussion of the disease. Many practitioners who served with McGrigor in Egypt also published accounts of their time there. These are important because they demonstrate that McGrigor's account cannot be taken at face value and, by contrasting with him, highlight the possibility that his efforts were intended to have a normative function. They also more directly acknowledge the importance of native and French practices on the development of British medicine in Egypt. Although these practitioners differed in their approach to the cure of the disease, they nearly all attributed the cause of it to the environment in which it was produced, Egypt. Interestingly, many also attempted to dissect that environment using the language and theoretical framework of chemistry. A high proportion of medical officers had undertaken some education at Edinburgh where chemistry was, by this time, one of the most popular courses.[83]

The starting point for this chemical analysis was probably based on Alpinus's 'nitrous salts' carried by the Egyptian winds. McGrigor was aware of this theory, however by using a process of elimination employed by many other practitioners to locate the source of this disease, he reasoned that while the salts, sand, heat and light of Egypt were 'existing' [*sic*] causes of the ophthalmia, they were all factors present in places where ophthalmia was not endemic, and therefore could not be its principal cause. In accordance with his preventative approach to health, he observed that officers were rarely affected by ophthalmia and concluded that cleanliness was essential to combat it. His first line of defence recommended the frequent washing of eyes and wearing something over them to protect them from the exciting causes of the disease. He then looked to written authority and attempted to apply Cullen's noseology to the ophthalmia and argued that it generally resolved into either of Cullen's two species, a combination of the two, or, thirdly, a species of ophthalmia frequent in India symptomatic of disease in the biliary secretion.

He considered the 'European practice' of scarification and astringent collyria but concluded it did not work in the first stage. He also noted that the natives used plant decoctions and poultices, frequent bathing of the eye in the last stage of the disease and often bled the patients. His recommendation for the 'best treatment' was similar to treatments generally adopted by the French: careful syringing of the patient's eyes with tepid filtered water for the first two to three days, the exclusion of light and heat and a strict antiphlogistic regime.[84] The next stage of treatment was a collyrium of a weak solution of sugar of lead or of camphor or vitriolated zinc. If the patient was in a lot of pain he recommended the addition of opium to the collyrium, and in the case of swelling, a saturine poultice.[85]

The surgeon Henry Dewar's views about medicine were deeply affected by his experiences in Egypt. On his return to Britain he wrote his doctoral dissertation on the Egyptian ophthalmia, and also published *Observations on Diarrhoea and Dysentery ... in the British Campaign of Egypt in 1801*.[86] In all his work he frequently referred to French authority, particularly to Savaresi, Larrey and Desgenettes. Their influence is also discernable in his association of ophthalmia with disordered states of the bowel and stomach and the suppression of 'customary evacuations'. In his later work, he stated that 'in Egypt, bowel complaints were observed by the medical gentlemen, both in the French service and ours, to alternate remarkably with ophthalmia'.[87]

Daniel Whyte held strong views on all the Egyptian diseases, not just the plague. In contrast to his opinions on the plague, his recommendations on the treatment of ophthamia and dysentery seem to have been widely disseminated and respected. His views on the Egyptian ophthalmia were published in the *Medical and Physical Journal* after his death.[88] The paper is in two parts, the first making a distinction between ordinary ocular inflammation (a result of an expansion of the humours and dilation of the eye's vessels on exposure to heat and light) and the Egyptian ophthalmia. In Egypt and Syria he believed there was a 'more pernicious source' of the disease: the particles of sand blown into the eye in the windy deserts. His recommended treatment was designed to 'second the efforts of Nature' by syringing the eye (mimicking the tear response) until the offending particles were removed. Once these particles were thus removed he merely continued with the treatment as for an ordinary inflammation. That treatment required the avoidance of heat and light and keeping the eye moist with a cloth dipped in cold water, or a gently astringent collyrium. He also found it useful to gently touch the ball of the eye with some astringent and stimulating tincture, such as cinchona or opium. In this first part of the paper he also urged strongly interventionist cures, such as the piercing of the eye to allow the humours to escape, and some bleeding, but in general was not in favour of scarification.

His paper is most interesting, however, because of its postscript in which he reveals that experience in Egypt had changed his mind about the efficacy of scarification, of which he began 'to think better ... and to practice ... oftener'. He also reports having been provided with the French works on ophthalmia by Sir Sydney Smith. His review of the works of the 'Franko-Egyptian' practitioners, Bruant and Savaresi, is quite negative because they were not advocates of scarification. He further argued that all the treatments the French identify are really just one common principle, 'stimulation'.

The practitioner to most closely investigate the link between climate and disease in Egypt was George Power.[89] Power dedicated his work to Thomas Young, in terms indicative of his extreme admiration for the man. His stated aims were to enquire into the contagiousness of ophthalmia, its connection with the plague and then to point out the different modes of treatment including those used by natives and the French surgeons and to contrast them with his own. Power's review of the published works on ophthalmia is comprehensive, drawing on Prosper Alpinus, Volney, Savaresi and the paper of Dr Whyte. Considering each of these authors in turn he used a process of elimination to discount their explanations for the cause of the disease. This process led him to deduce that the wide variety of opinions regarding the 'exciting and predisposing causes of the Egyptian Ophthalmia' revealed in fact that there was little understanding of it. Accordingly, he proposed instead to select the 'most rational' and reject others based on 'false principles or mere hypothetical conjectures'. Using this principle he rejected the sands of Egypt, the bright sun, diet, head shaving, the wearing of a turban and the French argillaceous earths as the 'efficient' cause of the disease (although admitting that any of them might be aggravating causes).[90] He then considered what Volney described as an 'unknown noxious quality' of the air in Egypt and concluded that the immense quantities of animal and vegetable substances in that country acted upon by the intense heat and moisture of the atmosphere could not fail but to pass into putrefactive fermentation. The absorption of this substance into the air, mixed with the earthy and saline substances of Egypt, he argued, through intricate chemical processes, and the contributions of insects, produced a malignant substance of 'foul and pestilent vapours under the generic term PUTRID VIRUS'.[91]

Power acknowledged that this same putrid virus must exist in other warm climates without producing the Egyptian diseases and concluded 'we must attribute the peculiarity of Egyptian diseases to some innate physical or moral causes, existing in the country itself, and constantly operating as one common predisposing cause'.[92] He then argued that the heat, too much bathing, excessive venery and immoderate use of tobacco and opium produced a corporeal and mental debility, the extensive sterile plain and the reflected light tortured the retina, and that sleeping at night in the open air led to the imbibing of the putrid virus from the dews. Interestingly, he argued that the extent of a person's debilitation would determine the effect of the putrid virus on the body, either producing ophthalmia in the eyes, in a more debilitated person, dysentery, and in the peculiarly debilitated, plague. Power saw the cause of these diseases of Egypt as being Egypt itself.[93]

His research in Egypt was extensive and he set out in detail the various treatments advocated by different writers and by the local inhabitants, but dismissed them all as ineffective. He stated that he discovered the best cure for the ophthalmia after catching it (in romantic style) himself:

> During this interval, being reduced to the lowest possible state of debility, one evening at sun-set, whilst looking at the distant Pyramids, I felt my eyes instantaneously suffused with a cold moist vapour, to which I had every reason afterwards to attribute the disease.[94]

He began to suffer from the ophthalmia the next day and tried several remedies but none were effective. As he was suffering a great deal of pain, he took opium which instead of sleepiness produced 'a degree of exhilaration', and when the pain returned he dosed himself again. In combination with occasional syringing to get rid of the discharge in his eyes, he found that opium cured the ophthalmia. He then used it on his fellow surgeon, Mr Davis who was also suffering and could not wait to give it to all the patients in his hospital: 'In the space of a month from the adoption of this remedy, we were enabled to restore to the Army almost every ophthalmic patient, in a state of convalescence or of perfect health'.[95]

Dysentery in Egypt

Power's identification of dysentery as one of the Egyptian diseases reflects its considerable incidence in Egypt, but it was generally acknowledged as a common, if deadly, military disease and would not initially have appeared 'new' to medical practitioners. However, the experience of dysentery in Egypt challenged the medical training of many of these gentlemen and many believed they were seeing it anew.

McGrigor's understanding of dysentery was changed by his experience in Egypt. He stated that his observations in Egypt made him question his previous beliefs about dysentery and the teachings of Cullen on the subject:

> The dysentery which occurred in the army till we came to the shores of the Mediterranean, and for some time after, was clearly the dysentery of India; but, afterwards, we witnessed a different disease. I must confess, that, having come to so certain a conclusion, I was not ready to give up an opinion which appeared to me to rest on very sure grounds; and it was not till after much doubt, hesitation, and careful observation, that I became convinced, in Alexandria, that, with the change of country and climate, we had a different disease.[96]

This revelation also confirmed McGrigor's belief, first formed during his West Indian service, that it was not possible to describe or know the disease of a particular climate without first hand observation: 'This is one proof of how improper, and how unsafe, it is for the practitioner of one climate to sit down and describe the diseases of another ... From reasoning of any kind, we are incompetent to decide on the identity of disease'.[97] His strenuous defence of the expertise of military practitioners for 'military diseases', examined in Chapter 6, was based on this philosophy.

Like McGrigor, Dewar stated that his observations of dysentery in Egypt forced him to question what he had been taught about the disease.[98] Dewar's treatment for dysentery was that recommended by Whyte and trialled successfully by McGrigor – swathing the abdomen in flannel. Dewar stated that Whyte had used the bandage with success in the Maltese corps hospital and had written a manuscript on the practice.[99] Dewar was keen to investigate the disease personally, but was unable to proceed with his preferred method, dissection, because he was working in a regimental hospital. He informed the reader that, 'as dissections, in the army, are chiefly confined to general hospitals, and meet with opposition in regimental practice, I had no opportunity of examining in this matter, the effects of [dysentery]' instead he had to turn to local practices and the works of Pringle, Morgagni and Hunter.[100]

Like his colleagues, Dewar ultimately attributed the diseases of the Egyptian campaign to the enervating effects of the hot climate on Europeans.[101] This core belief also drove McGrigor's approach to Egypt. His account of his time in

Egypt sets out his routine in the recording daily information about the weather, his experiments to determine the amount of dew falling overnight, and his belief that not only the change in seasons, but also the sol-lunar influence, was important to the onset of disease. He stated 'I am decidedly of the opinion, that in the peculiar soil and climate of Egypt we are to look for the principal causes of the diseases which prevailed the most in that country'.[102] Summing up the Egyptian investigations he stated that 'On two particulars a good deal of time has been paid, as well as attention; namely, the state of the weather and the dissections of the dead',[103] for him, the beginning and end of disease.

The importance attributed to the Egyptian environment as the primary cause of plague, ophthalmia and dysentery on the campaign by nearly all the British military medical officers was shaken by the appearance of an Egyptian ophthalmia epidemic amongst British troops several years after the army returned home, and questions were raised about the nature of the disease. Theories that favoured dirt, disorder and contagion as the cause of the ophthalmia achieved wide acceptance amongst military practitioners, but civilian practitioners challenged the distinctness of the disorder and the relevance of overseas service to treating it.

Ophthalmia in Britain

The French and British works on the Egyptian campaign were published soon after the return of the armies from Egypt. As McGrigor stated, 'Egypt and Arabia peculiarly interest[ed] every man of science, and more particularly medical men, from the occurrence of the plague, and the ophthalmia, in Egypt'.[104] The interest of military and civilian practitioners in these works became heightened when an epidemic of ophthalmia swept through the armies of Europe. Fears were expressed that it would soon infect 'the lower orders of society' and from thence, everyone. Egyptian ophthalmia was carried to their home countries by each of the armies that had served in Egypt, and in Britain was responsible for the invaliding of thousands of soldiers, whole regiments of whom had never been in Egypt.[105] The problem soon came to be perceived as not only medically, but also politically, important. The troops suffering from ophthalmia were needed to fight the Wars and were costing the State thousands of pounds in pensions. Army practitioners continued to use many of the treatments that had been developed in Egypt, and innovations also emerged.[106] A characteristic of these new treatments was their association with particular individuals. In 1808 and 1809, the epidemic became particularly severe and, in the context of an existing manpower crisis facing the forces, prompted influential army officers and politicians to turn their attention to the disease, ultimately prompting a bitter dispute between civilian and military practitioners over the 'territory' of ophthalmia.

The progression of attitudes to the ophthalmia, can be tracked in the publications which began to appear a few years after the return of the troops. The problem facing practitioners was that a disease which had been so closely linked with Egypt's climate was thriving in a very different environment. Accordingly, the issue to which many physicians addressed themselves was the nature of the disease, particularly whether it arose not from the environment but from contagion.

Arthur Edmonston was a surgeon with the 2nd Regiment of the Argyleshire Fencibles. He wrote a pamphlet in 1802 describing his experience of ophthalmia in the regiment, and argued that the disease was contagious.[107] Ophthalmia had appeared amongst his regiment when it travelled from Gibraltar to Spithead on board a ship which had served in Egypt. Edmonston investigated the disease by writing to the other Fencible regiments who had been stationed at Gibraltar at the same time and those surgeons wrote back indicating that the ophthalmia 'prevailed very generally amongst them'.[108] He also found on returning to Gibraltar that the regiments which had subsequently been stationed there 'had all been in Egypt, and had all suffered more or less from Ophthalmia' and that it had spread amongst the local population.[109] These facts, in addition to his own observations convinced Edmonston of the contagiousness of ophthalmia. He asserted that the British practitioners returning from Egypt were 'unwilling to give in to the idea that the Ophthalmia which prevailed there was contagious'.[110] In 1806, he produced his *Treatise on Ophthalmia* which focused strongly on the contagiousness of the disease and sought to prove it by tracking the progression of ophthalmia through regiments in contact with each other. He also tried to provide an explanation of the method of transmission.

Edmonston gave much credit to the works of the practitioners who had been stationed in Egypt, particularly the works of the French, especially Bruant. It is clear that he was very familiar with, and had great respect for, these works. He was also familiar with Dewar's dissertation. However, Edmonston believed that practitioners in Egypt had missed the contagious nature of the disease because of the dramatic and filthy environment in which they had encountered it: 'when so many obvious sources of irritation prevail, the discriminating shades elude our perception, and prevent the attainment of that precision of arrangement, and accuracy of information, so desirable in every philosophical research'.[111] Edmonston argued that:

> since the Ophthalmia of Egypt ... became the object of general observation, several medical men have been induced to change their views of the subject; and begin to believe that a disease which has hitherto been considered as purely local, is often propagated by contagion.[112]

He thought that the contagion could be passed simply by sleeping in the same room as an infected person, or close proximity to their eye. In particular, he thought that the discharge from the eyes was particularly dangerous, having the ability to get into bedding and clothes, and thereby becoming more easily spread than the contagion operating through the air which only had a reach of approximately one foot. He pondered deeply on the very nature of contagion in his work. The analogy first made by Larrey between ophthalmia and gonorrhoea may have influenced Edmonston in this regard, and he referred, as did many practitioners on the subject of contagious ophthalmia, to the infection of the natives of Tahiti with venereal disease. [113]

His recommended treatment for ophthalmia was very different to that proposed by McGrigor, and perhaps reflected fashions that developed after his return from Egypt. He recommended the use of 'topical blood-letting' by the 'division of the vessels on the conjunctiva and eyeball' but warned that it was imperative to perform this operation at exactly the right stage of the disease. In discussing the difficulty of that evaluation he revealed that his method was not the preferred cure amongst his colleagues in Egypt: 'The difficulty of making a nice discrimination in this respect appears to me one great reason why so many medical gentlemen in Egypt were adverse to the use of scarification'. [114] However, as will be seen later in this chapter, his practice was very similar to that adopted by many practitioners in Britain after the campaign.

Dr John Vetch came into contact with the ophthalmia when his regiment, the 52nd of light infantry, was stationed at Hythe. He was to become one of the most prominent men in the conflict over the 'territory' of ophthalmia after the Wars discussed in Chapter 6. In 1807, he published *An Account of the Ophthalmia which has Appeared in England since the Return of the British Army from Egypt*. He began by positioning himself as one of the 'moderns' dedicated to observation and experience:

> as the properties of the thing examined should always be first ascertained, before inquiring into its relations, the reader, will, perhaps, be as well pleased to find the number of following pages not augmented by extracts from the writings of Avicenna or Albucasis. [115]

He then gave an account of the extremely violent and destructive nature of the ophthalmia in England:

> The total strength of the second battalion of the 52nd... was somewhat above seven hundred men: six hundred and thirty six cases of ophthalmia, including relapses, were admitted into the hospital, from August 1805, when the disease commenced, till the same month in 1806; of these fifty were dismissed with the loss of both eyes, and forty with that of one. [116]

Vetch believed that this was the same disease as that which had attacked the troops in Egypt, and sought to prove that connection by tracking the movements of men from barrack to barrack, finally pinpointing Irish soldiers who had joined his troops after serving in regiments garrisoned with men who had suffered ophthalmia in Egypt. The point Vetch was seeking to make was that the disease was contagious and transmitted by the discharge from the eyes of the infected.[117] In this respect he drew an analogy with the specific matter of contagion in gonorrhoea, possibly drawing on the suspicions of Larrey. The most alarming thing about the disease for Vetch was that it was 'capable of propagating itself independent of any peculiarity of climate'.[118] However, he did think that climate was relevant to the aggravation of the disease and that the ophthalmia was much worse in England than it had been in Egypt.[119]

Vetch considered the appropriate treatment for ophthalmia, and recorded a series of experiments with mild bloodletting, local applications, the use of cold, neutral salts, solutions of opium, warm applications, mercury and cinchona.[120] Despite the generally prevailing opinion amongst authors, both ancient and modern, 'that purgatives have been the most recommended as a remedy superior to almost every other', he found that they yielded little benefit, although emetics did offer some relief. The portrait painted by Vetch of his attempts to cure the disease is rather hopeless. However, this bleak outlook changed upon the 'heroic intervention' of the inspector general of army hospitals, Francis Knight, in May 1806.

Vetch reports that Knight came to investigate what was happening in the 52nd and, to treat the disease, 'laid down plans no less decisive in themselves, than successful in their issue'.[121] Knight decided that the hospital should be kept for ophthalmia patients alone, and that all those suspected of having ophthalmia should be removed to separate barracks, he also created barracks solely for convalescents arranged according to the severity and stage of their infection. But Knight's most insightful directive was as follows:

> The urgent nature of the disease, and the inefficacy of the previous treatment, demanded the most active measures; but at the same time it required much professional knowledge to guide them, Notwithstanding the undisturbed state of the system, and apparently in opposition to the experience which had been already gained, Mr Knight proposed the most decided antiphlogistic regimen, with the regular exhibition of purgatives, and above all the use of the lancet, with a freedom far beyond what had been formerly thought of.[122]

Knight's solution, which Vetch states worked very well, was to bleed the patient to the point of syncope (fainting). Despite the seemingly drastic nature of this cure it was reported, with apparent approval, in the *Edinburgh Medical and Surgical Journal*.[123]

Vetch believed that Knight's plan would cure many afflicted soldiers, but still feared that it would be impossible to prevent the spread of the disease to the lower classes of society, and from there to society in general. He thought that the only real solution to the problem was to prevent the disease. In proposing practical measures to prevent the spread of the disease Vetch restricted himself to the field in which he felt he could speak with authority – the army. By doing so he unwittingly presaged the debate in which he was to become embroiled, on the competence of civilian and military practitioners to treat ophthalmia. The practical advice he offered was simple and suited to military culture, a daily and minute inspection by the medical officers and supervision by an officer while the men washed their faces and eyes from separate bowls of water.[124]

In 1807, George Peach, also a surgeon of the 52nd foot, wrote to McGrigor, now deputy inspector general of hospitals, about Knight's cure.[125] Peach told how he had first unsuccessfully attempted an antiphlogistic regime, and then trialled Peruvian Bark and other stimulants to treat ophthalmia. Only after these also proved ineffectual (with 733 cases including relapses out of a strength of 691) did Peach try an antiphlogistic treatment 'in its fullest extent'. His letter records his own surprise at his success, 'This practice, I fancy, would astonish the experience of civil life, but the fullest trial of it has demonstrated to me its propriety'.[126]

The distinction between civilian and military practice was echoed from across the divide by Dr James Ware, a civilian practitioner, who warned that even though the depletion treatment had been very successful in the army, 'it is necessary ... to make an allowance for the difference that is to be expected between a disorder in a military hospital, and one, similar to it, in private practice'. He had adopted Knight's treatment but found moderate bleeding to be sufficient in his civilian practice.[127]

McGrigor demonstrated his attachment to the centralization of information, and took it upon himself to forward Peach's letter to the *Edinburgh Medical and Surgical Journal*, stating it was, 'an account of a disease, which is daily extending its ravages through the army, and, if not checked, may cripple our navy and army, this statement cannot be too widely or quickly diffused'.[128] He lent his support to Knight's bleeding treatment by adding, 'The practice, at length so successfully had recourse to by Mr Peach and Dr Vetch in the 52nd regiment, has, I know, been eminently successful in other quarters, particularly by Mr Reid in the 89th regiment, and by Mr Waugh in the 8th Veteran Battalion'.[129] In a second letter Peach stated that he had recommended the treatment to other surgeons and that it had done well. In that letter he also hastened to point out that he and Vetch tried everything else before resorting to this desperate measure:

in the ophthalmia of Egypt, which I have been so much engaged in for two years, during which time I have had, in the 52nd regiment, 1341 cases under my care, I may be
allowed to decide on venesection being the sovereign remedy for this disease: it is not
because I have not had recourse to other means; there are, indeed, few remedies I had
not resorted to, and given up as useless of inefficacious, before Dr. Vetch and myself
had recourse to venesection.[130]

McGrigor lent an even stronger endorsement to the treatment on this occasion,
stating, 'The cure of intermittents by bark, and of syphilis by mercury, is not
more certain than the successful treatment of the Egyptian Ophthalmia by the
method here recommended by Mr Peach'.[131]

The success of this method and the involvement of Mr Knight were also
reported in other medical journals:

> The aggravated violence of its symptoms has now been judiciciously met at last, by
> pursuing a system of depletion, carried to an extreme. The lancet has been used to
> an excess, with the most fortunate issue; and the disease has been suspended in the
> progress of its first ravages, by the abstraction of 30, 40, or even 60 ounces of blood,
> and thus prevented from passing on to its secondary and dangerous stage. The merit
> of this improvement is due to Mr. Knight, the Inspector-General, who has justly pro-
> portioned his measures with adequate energy, to the activity of the morbid cause.[132]

The efforts of men like Knight and McGrigor to standardize the treatment for
ophthalmia culminated in the issuing of directions on the treatment of this disease by the inspector general. The treatment, designed to counter the extreme
inflammation of the first stages of the disease, appears to have been widely
adopted. Hirschberg states that 'bloodletting until unconsciousness occurs,
again bleeding and once again using the lancet with extraordinary boldness' was
the gospel preached between 1804 and 1818, and remained a popular practice
for many years after, only being comprehensively rejected in 1860.[133] The most
graphic, and enthusiastic, account of the treatment was given by Dr Charles
Farrell, who had worked under Dr Franklin in the ophthalmic army hospital in
Sicily between 1808 and 1810.[134] He also commented that most of the failures
to cure the disorder were the result of taking the advice of civilian doctors who,
while generally very skilled, really had no idea about the violence of the ophthalmia because they had not seen it for themselves.[135]

It was not possible, despite these efforts, to completely standardize the
approach of surgeons to this disorder. In the same edition of the *Edinburgh Medical and Surgical Journal*, which contained Knight and McGrigor's best efforts
to promote the bleeding treatment, C. F. Forbes, surgeon of the 4th Battalion
of the Royals in Edinburgh Castle, reported his success with scarification using
a straight blade developed by James Wardrop instead of the common lancet.[136]

Conflicting ideas about the nature of the disease were also being expressed. Many drew on the connection between ophthalmia and venereal disease identified by Larrey. These ideas questioned the 'newness' of the ophthalmia, and can be seen partly as an attempt by civilian practitioners to prevent military practitioners asserting special experience of, or skill with, the disease. Dr Ware, challenged the idea that the ophthalmia spreading among the troops was the same as the Egyptian ophthalmia. He argued that exactly the same ophthalmia had previously been described by ancient and modern authors in England as well as other countries. He insisted that it was best to call the current epidemic 'purulent ophthalmy' based on its distinguishing symptom of purulent discharge. The resemblance he perceived between this ophthalmia and the ophthalmia which accompanies or follows gonorrhoea, gave him the strong impression that those 'two disorders bear a close reference to each other'.[137] His argument was taken up in an anonymous pamphlet 'Identities Ascertained', in which the author ultimately concluded that the same disease could have its 'seat' in different organs in different parts of the world.[138]

The 'newness' of the disease was also questioned in the *Surgical Spectator*:

> This epidemic Ophthalmia, which has created so much mischief in our armies, has given scope to the pens of a number of our military practitioners, and we give them credit for their attempts to elucidate its nature and treatment. But, like every subject in vogue, the Egyptian ophthalmia has been seen where it never existed, and obstinate cases of the common ophthalmia of this country it is now fashionable to refer to an Egyptian source. The Egyptian ophthalmia is chiefly distinguished by its enormous quantity of purulent discharge; but although purulencey is an attendant of severe cases in this country, it is not to be supposed the same identical disease. These hints we merely throw out to caution practitioners against referring to a new origin what is a common disease of this climate.[139]

To complicate matters a second epidemic of 'ophthalmia' was spreading amongst the troops, 'malingering ophthalmia'. Soldiers in the 28th Regiment of foot were discovered putting substances in their eyes to produce a high degree of ocular inflammation thus exempting them from duty and possibly resulting in a discharge from the army. Vetch wrote about this 'epidemic' and was evidently concerned that the practice had undermined belief in the real Egyptian ophthalmia. To assist medical officers he set out the differences between the two afflictions hoping to forestall the belief that the Egyptian ophthalmia did not exist in Britain.[140]

Debates over the nature of the ophthalmia, its origin or reality, carried on while the disease continued its ravages in Britain. Towards the end of 1807, three hospital wards were created for ophthalmic patients at the depot in Bognor and Dr Vetch was appointed as the commanding officer. In the summer of 1808, he had charge of 900 patients from 40 different army corps.[141] In August 1808, Mr

Keate, the surgeon general, wrote to the secretary at war, requesting he and the commander-in-chief, 'devise means ... for arresting [the ophthalmia's] progress'. Keate suggested the creation of a Board to investigate:

> the best means of accomplishing this important object ... and which Board may consist of such members, besides the Army Medical Board, as may be deemed competent by their attainments and experience, to so important an inquiry.[142]

This suggestion was taken up, and in 1810 a Board was appointed. The Board included the three members of the AMB, and eight others, all civilian practitioners. The suggestions of this civilian-dominated Board, which concentrated on prevention through cleanliness, were then circulated to army medical officers in general orders from the Horse Guards.[143] Unfortunately, the ophthalmia epidemic was not arrested by the measures recommended. As will be discussed in Chapter 6, throughout the following decade military and civilian practitioners, backed by their political patrons, engaged in a bitter and personal dispute over the right to treat, and the best treatment for, the growing number of ophthalmic pensioners.

Conclusion

The Egyptian environment was entirely new to French and British military practitioners in a way that the exotic environments of India and the West Indies were not at this time. Egypt occupied a place in literature as the cradle of civilization as well as the cradle of disease. Previously, only the most adventurous practitioners like Alpinus and Whyte had been drawn to the region. The French, and after them the British, approached the 'new diseases' of Egypt not primarily by turning to theory, but instead to practical measures: segregation followed by experimentation. They tried almost anything, and were interested in, if not enthusiastic about, the cures used by local people. Their experiment and observation extended beyond the patient to the environment in which they were operating. The extremes they faced, the traumas they suffered and their empirical observations led British military practitioners to believe that only by going through those processes could these diseases really be understood. The aberrant behaviour of dysentery in Egypt confirmed this notion.

The campaign was also significant in the development of McGrigor's approach to the command of a medical corps, and allowed him to implement processes which both collated new information about disease and embedded him at the centre of a knowledge network. Over the course of the rest of the Wars, McGrigor attempted to use this process to erode independence of practice within the medical department by promoting particular approaches and therapies. His knack for weaving together medical measures and military priorities was further demonstrated on this campaign and led him to define medical success in terms of prevention.

The epidemic of ophthalmia that spread to Britain gave military medical practitioners the opportunity to apply the knowledge they had gathered overseas in the domestic environment. However, the appearance of a 'foreign disease' on home shores prompted a re-thinking of the nature of the ophthalmia and helped to promote filth and contagion models over climatic theories of disease. Through debates about the nature of the disease, and the therapies that should be used to treat it, the seeds of discord between military and civilian practitioners were sown.

4 THE PENINSULAR WAR

The following two chapters consider the Peninsular War and demonstrate how and why army medicine and army medical officers became increasingly militarized. In particular, the implications for the development of army medicine resulting from the appointment of the new AMB are discussed. By examining the relative success and failure of the most senior military medical officers, the chapters highlight how important it had become for medical officers to adapt their practice to accommodate not only the practicalities of campaigning, but also the values of army culture.

The Peninsular War, a series of campaigns over six years from 1808 to 1814, was precipitated by Napoleon's movement of 100,000 troops into Spain with the intention of invading Portugal. The ensuing Spanish rebellion and Portuguese resistance provided the British government with the necessary allies and motivation to mount a campaign on the Continent, and an expeditionary force of 13,000 men under Sir Arthur Wellesley set sail for Portugal in July 1808. Following reports of a larger French presence in Portugal, the British force was increased to 40,000 men, and the command given to Sir Hew Dalrymple, with Sir Henry Burrard as his deputy. Those gentlemen arrived in Portugal after Wellesley's victories at Roliça and Vimeiro, just in time to prevent an advance and secure the much-regretted Convention of Cintra that allowed the French to evacuate Portugal. The subsequent departure of Wellesley, Dalrymple and Burrard left Sir John Moore at the head of a British army of 30,000 men. With the arrival of Napoleon in the Peninsula, Moore's leadership was to end with a disastrous retreat westwards across Portugal, culminating in the evacuation of the army from Corunna to England in January 1809. British troops returned to the Peninsula that April, once again under the command of Wellesley, and remained there over several campaigning seasons until word came of Napoleon's defeat while the British army were engaged at Toulouse in 1814.[1]

Perhaps owing to the numerous personal accounts of the Peninsular War that were published after the peace which gave lurid accounts of 'amputation hospitals' and the horrors of battlefield medicine, British involvement in the Peninsular War has received more attention from medical historians than any other campaign of the Wars. In particular, the retreat from Corunna and the latter campaigns of the Duke of Wellington (1812–14) have been extensively researched.[2] The Peninsular War is usually seen as significant because of the reforms and achievements of James McGrigor while at the head of the service from 1812 to1814, and most medical histories of the period focus on him, taking as their guide his own account of the campaigns.[3] However, McGrigor's tenure was actually shorter than that of his predecessor, Dr James Franck, who headed the medical department from 1808, returning to England as an invalid in the summer of 1811.

Meticulous details of the administrative arrangements of the medical department under both Franck and McGrigor, military aspects of each campaign and the diseases encountered by the army as it moved around the region are provided by Cantlie who divides his consideration of the Peninsular War into two chronological sections: the first from 1808 to 1811; and the second from 1812 to 1814. Although he does not characterize it as such, his dividing point is clearly the arrival of McGrigor. Cantlie's division reflects the bulk of medical histories of the Peninsular War that present a narrative in which McGrigor is the hero of the piece, supported by George Guthrie as the swashbuckling hero of the surgical field.[4] This concentration on McGrigor, and the repetition of almost set-piece tales to emphasize his importance, has unfortunately detracted from a fuller examination of the medical history of the Peninsular War, both by de-emphasizing what can be learned from the years before McGrigor's arrival, and by stifling re-examination of the documents relevant to McGrigor's tenure outside the well-worn track followed by most historians in the footsteps of Cantlie.

Despite the long period in which Franck was the inspector of hospitals under Wellington, he is usually given short shrift, and although not often criticized, always damned with faint praise. Cantlie says only that, 'it is not to decry the ability of Dr. Franck when we say that with McGrigor's appearance on the scene a new era began for the Medical department in the Peninsula'.[5] While, Blanco comments, 'one looks in vain at Franck's tenure of office for a single major improvement'.[6] Similarly, the British medical force seconded to the Portuguese army, headed by Dr William Fergusson, although routinely mentioned by historians, has never been properly examined, despite the continued availability of all Fergusson's official papers. Fergusson's efforts to reform the Portuguese medical department are noted by most historians as a success, but little further analysis is undertaken.[7]

The 'McGrigor years' in the Peninsula will be examined in the following chapter. This chapter will investigate the effects of the Corunna retreat on the AMD, as well as considering the importance of Franck's and Fergusson's experiences in the Peninsula prior to 1812, and their relevance to the ongoing medical debates arising from the preceding campaigns of the Wars.

Corunna

One of the most notorious events of the Wars was the retreat from Sagahun to Corunna undertaken by Sir John Moore's army in the winter of 1808. Moore had been left in charge of a force of 30,000 men in Lisbon after Dalrymple, Burrard and Wellesley were called back to Britain. Following the arrival of Sir David Baird's force of 14,000 men at Corunna in October 1808, Moore decided to take 20,000 of his men and rendezvous with Baird. He intended that they would advance into Spain and assist the Spanish in driving out the remaining French. Moore's intended meeting point was Valladolid in northern Spain – a significant journey from either Lisbon or Corunna, over difficult and mountainous terrain. Moore and Baird advanced into Spain, but before they could attack the French, Moore received intelligence of Napoleon's arrival in the country at the head of a very significant force. To preserve Britain's army, Moore was forced to order an urgent retreat to Corunna on the coast. Once arrived at Corunna, the ragged and exhausted army were obliged to engage in a battle with the pursuing French, and despite winning a victory, suffered the loss of its leader when Moore was mortally wounded. [8]

Many first-hand accounts of the retreat across Spain and Portugal were published shortly after the army returned to England. They paint a uniformly horrific picture, replete with evocative descriptions of the horrors suffered, particularly by the women and children who accompanied the army. Dr Adam Neale who wrote to his friends from several places along the retreat, and later published those letters, drew a common sketch:

> Broken wagons and carriages, money-carts, dead animals, and the bodies of human beings, who had perished from the inclemency of the weather during the night, strewed the way for miles. Never had I conceived, much less witnessed, so awful a scene. [9]

Neale's is the only detailed account of the retreat written by a medical officer, and his letters demonstrate the difficulties he encountered in procuring (and retaining) wagons to transport the sick over whom he was given charge, [10] establishing them in hospitals at each stop, and his efforts to keep his convoy separated from the sick of the allied Spanish army who had, 'in addition to their other misfortunes, a most malignant typhus fever raging amongst their troops'. [11] Neale blamed contact with that Spanish army for the typhus that was to wreak such destruction on the British. [12] The conditions experienced by the armies as they raced back to the coast with the French nipping at their heels, unfortunately encouraged the spread of the disease. Onboard the crowded transports that took the sick from Corunna to England; the louse that carried the disease thrived:

> For two days after we came on board, I felt the most severe pains throughout my whole body: the change was so great, from the extreme cold of the winter nights,

which we had passed almost without covering, to the suffocating heat of a crowded transport. This was not the most disagreeable part: vermin began to abound. We had not been without them on our march: but now we had dozens for one we had then. In vain we killed them; they appeared to increase from the ragged and dirty clothes, of which we had no means of freeing ourselves. Complaint was vain. Many were worse than myself.[13]

The imminent return of these beleaguered troops to England sparked alarm amongst the AMB, owing to the closure of the general hospitals at Portsmouth, Gosport, and Deal by Francis Knight (discussed in Chapter 2).[14] Of a force of 34,000 men, nearly 4,000 had been lost on the campaign and a further 4,305 were listed as sick on the arrival of the army in England.[15] The efforts of McGrigor (then deputy inspector of the South West District) to secure accommodation for what he termed 'the wreck of our unfortunate army from Spain'[16] in the naval hospital at Haslar, and in barracks and various ships anchored at Spithead, only narrowly avoided an even greater crisis.

The medical crisis occasioned by the Corunna disaster provides a fitting entrée to the developments in the army medical service that were to unfold over the following six years. Within the responses to it can be seen the beginnings of several very important themes: the active promotion of the idea that 'on-the-field' training could be more valuable than university learning; the incorporation of military ideals into medical theory, particularly by McGrigor; and the particular style McGrigor used in his efforts to standardize clinical practice among army medical officers.

The massive influx of sick required more medical assistance than the AMD could provide from within its own ranks and pleas were made by Francis Knight to the medical schools of the country for students to volunteer as hospital mates for the duration of the crisis. One such student, William Dent, wrote to his mother:

> Mr. Ashley Cooper [*sic*] the Surgeon and Lecturer at St. Thomas Hospital, has received a letter from Mr. Knight, the Inspector of Hospitals, desiring all the Students that possibly can leave town, for to go to different districts to attend and dress the Sick and wounded soldiers that have arrived from Spain ... Mr Cooper hoped that every young man that could go would, for he looked upon it both as humanity and as a duty to do so at such an emergency, he said that they would have that practice which it was impossible they could see at present in London, as it would be only of a temporary nature, not exceeding a Month or six weeks, he trusted that it would not interrupt our studies.[17]

Dent responded to the call and found himself working with the Battalion of the 4th Regiment at Colchester in which there were 'one hundred and ninety seven Men sick and wounded in the Hospital, and half of this number I have to take care of myself'. He agreed with Cooper's prediction that it would be a valuable learning experience, 'I am very glad that I came here for besides attending the Sick and wounded, we have the privilege of dissecting those who die, and in London we could not get a dead Body under three guineas'.[18] But contrary to expectations, he was not to return to his official studies within 'six weeks', and continued to be attached to the Regiment for nearly a year, only returning to his studies in January. He was soon to come back to the army, passing his examination at the Royal College of Surgeons in May, and then the AMB.[19] On being sent to Hilsea Barracks near Portsmouth, he wrote to his mother (who had hoped he would settle in private practice):

> I hope you don't fret at my entering the Army. I am perfectly happy, and I see no rea-son why you should not be so, for I think the Army an excellent School for a young man, who has a desire to excel either in his profession or to become acquaint'd with the manners of the World.[20]

Dent's experience was common to many young men studying medicine towards the start of the Peninsular War, and his enthusiasm for the life it offered him is evident in his letters home. The notion that his experience with the Regiment was at least as beneficial as his formal studies is implicit not only in his repeti-tion of Cooper's statement that it would be so, but also in his assertions of the opportunities available to him for dissection with the army, and in his statement to his mother, not long after returning to London, that he believed he was ready to be examined.[21] As discussed in earlier chapters, this belief was central to a 'military medical identity', and had been expressed by leaders within the army medical community. At this time, it appears that the idea was taken up by a new cohort of recruits, engaged by the army during the vast expansion of the medical department during the Peninsular War, to justify their career choices.[22] Dent's experience helps us to see how the demand for hospital mates, the excitement of regimental life and the tangible difference between a dry lecture theatre and a vast hospital of sick, would have combined to support his ready adoption of that perspective on the value of 'on-the-field' experience.[23]

Men like Dent would not have found themselves short of hands-on expe-rience among the returned army. The *Edinburgh Medical and Surgical Journal* published two accounts of the sick returned from Corunna by medical officers who attended them, one in 1809 by Richard Hooper, a military surgeon,[24] and the second in 1810 by McGrigor. Both indicated that the prevailing diseases were dysentery and fever, and went into some detail on the treatments used to combat the diseases.

Hooper's account of his struggle to treat the dysentery affecting the troops is reminiscent of the process used by medical officers during the Egyptian cam-paign. Although dysentery was a common disease amongst armies, the virulence of the post-Corunna epidemic perplexed him and he treated it, in effect, like a 'new' disease. He began by using emetics and purgatives but:

> flattering as were the effects of these medicines, I soon found that no hopes of curing the complaint could be reasonably entertained ... [and] baffled in my attempts to relieve these miserable beings, I determined to see what a more general use of evacuants would do.[25]

He was later induced by the senior medical officer at his hospital to try acetate of lead by mouth, but also to no avail. In his final reckoning 'Having tried emetics, purgatives, the pulv. ipecac. comp. aromatics, calomel, the starch injection, acetate of lead, and opium to a certain extent'.[26] nothing was useful in curing the disease. His practice in treating typhus does not appear to have been much more successful, despite a similar variety of treatments.

McGrigor's paper, in which he collated reports from all the medical officers serving under him during the crisis, confirms the ubiquity of Hooper's experience. In keeping with the style he employed during the Egyptian campaign, McGrigor appears to have been trying to operate as a 'hub' and disseminator of medical information on a disease that was defying medical treatment.

McGrigor's paper focuses on the symptoms and treatment of fever, rather than dysentery. His overview shows that, in this disease also, a wide variety of treatments were tried including cordials and stimulants, bleeding and evacuations, mercury and cold affusion. He stated that 'the treatment ... varied very much with the different practitioners', but argued that this was because 'the varied form in which the disease appeared called for this variety in practice'.[27] Despite McGrigor's justification of the varying treatments used, it is clear that, at this time, army medical practitioners (at least those at the head of their own regimental or general hospitals) had enormous discretion in their medical practice, and were only subject to orders in the conduct of the sanitary part of the running of their departments. As will be demonstrated in the following chapter, at the head of the service in the Peninsula, McGrigor extended the reach of his self-appointed 'dissemination' role and attempted to standardize clinical practice throughout the army.[28] Probably owing to the tradition of clinical independence amongst military medics, McGrigor often tried to achieve this end through covert methods, some of which are apparent in this account of the Corunna sick. He was assiduous in mentioning the names of each practitioner, and in heaping praise upon their efforts. However, in his thorough account of the practices used to treat the fever, he made the following comment about Mr Burnett, the surgeon in charge of the hospitals for prisoners of war in the area: 'Mr Burnett's authority is of considerable weight. The prisoners of war here are seldom under 10,000; and in the hospitals under Mr Burnett there are seldom fewer than 300 sick.'[29]

By highlighting Burnett's practice in this way and specifically by attributing a 'weighting' to his 'authority', McGrigor tacitly endorsed Burnett's use of liberal evacuations and bleeding in the early stages of the disease. McGrigor's attribution of Burnett's 'weight' to his attendance on large numbers of sick in one place also emphasized the type of evidence McGrigor considered should be probative in deciding medical questions – first-hand experience in the treatment of large populations.

McGrigor's paper also reveals a great deal about the way in which he was incorporating military and political expediencies into his 'theory of disease' and his medical publications. Early in his account McGrigor attributed the cause of the illness to overtly military factors: the dispirited feelings of the army, and the disintegration of 'order and discipline, so necessary to its health', in addition to more 'medical' causes like their lack of clothing on a winter retreat and their contact with the infected Spanish army. He also stated that the medical situation of the army was made even worse by its being conveyed on poorly ventilated and unclean ships, on which many were obliged to stay for an extended period because of bad weather at Portsmouth and Plymouth. McGrigor was very pointed in labelling these major causes of the disease 'misfortunes', and suggesting that there was no utility in dwelling upon them.

His account was also extremely defensive of the medical officers, both for their medical competencies, and for their military valour, stating 'theirs was a service of as real danger as any that had occurred to military officers in Spain'.[30] In the course of this defence of the medical department, McGrigor was also sure to point out that the entire heroic effort had been orchestrated by 'Mr Knight, the Inspector-General'.[31] In this section of McGrigor's work we can see his articulation of key parts of the 'military medical identity' – a medicine designed to reinforce the importance of military discipline, practised by medical officers with excellent abilities, and which strongly identified the 'militarism' of medical officers outside their purely medical role. The political reasons for McGrigor's very defensive tone and comment on such matters in what was, ostensibly, a scientific and medical record of an epidemic, become clear when the serious allegations that were made by military medical officers, and by parliamentarians, about the care of the Corunna men are considered.

Following the return of the army, questions about the medical care provided both in the Peninsula and in England were raised by medical officers who had been present, and those complaints became the subject of a military inquiry. The nature of those complaints, and the structure and investigative approach of the inquiry reveal much about the militarization of medical officers and the concerns of military medical officers themselves.

Shortly after the army returned, several medical officers who had served with Sir John Moore wrote to the AMB expressing criticisms of the way in which the medical department had been conducted both in the Peninsula and throughout the evacuation. As mentioned in Chapter 2, Lucas Pepys and Thomas Keate seized upon these letters to bolster their argument against the use of regimental hospitals at the expense of general hospitals, advocated by their fellow board member and enemy, Francis Knight. In a letter to Sir James Pulteney, the secretary at war, Pepys and Keate stated that the reports of Adam Neale and Charles Tice 'demonstrate the horrors if the system of Regimental Hospitals on foreign service is to be — persevered in to supersede the use of General Hospitals'.[32]

In his letter, Neale had commented negatively on both the arrangements of Dr. Shapter (the head of the medical services of Moore's army) and on those in Portsmouth, both for the same reason: their being run on the regimental plan.[33] Charles Tice was less vitriolic but also complained that the mortality among the troops would have been greatly lessened if they had been housed in general hospitals on their return.[34] A similar letter was written by A. B. Faulkner criticizing the arrangements for the sick whilst awaiting evacuation from Corunna, and the exacerbation of their illness owing to the closure of the general hospitals in England.[35] Finally, Edward Knight, physician to the forces, also wrote to state that the accommodation for the returned sick in Ramsgate had been hopelessly crowded and that, 'Had these men been placed in the large and airy wards of our General Hospitals the spreading of the disorder would have been prevented and the mortality confined to a very small number'.

To support his position, Knight tendered the evidence that Major General Hope had inspected the hospital and 'after examining all its parts observed that it was the worst Hospital he had ever seen'.[36] Parliamentarians must also have been made aware of similar criticisms, as complaints about the medical care given to the army were raised in Parliament.[37]

Francis Knight requested that the papers be submitted to the commander-in-chief.[38] David Dundas laid the matter before the King, who commanded him to assemble a Board of General Officers for 'the purpose of taking the whole matter into consideration and reporting their opinion thereupon'.[39] That Board entirely comprised military officers, but the matters they investigated were purely medical.[40] The report they produced was over twenty pages long and extremely detailed. They investigated the management of Dr Shapter's hospital in Salamanca and the care and diet given to the men, finding:

> every possible attention was given by Doctor Shapter and Mr Warran to the due care of the sick at Salamanca and that tho' it be true, that irregularities did arise there which ought as far as possible to be prevented and which it is therefore fit to have reported and made known, yet we must observe that in the letters transmitted to us

much more importance has been given to those circumstances, than upon a careful examination the case seems either to have required or to warrant.[41]

In the course of their investigation of other complaints regarding the condition of the transports, speed of disembarkation of the sick, and care of the sick once arrived back in England, the Board of General Officers examined various medical and military officers. In its findings, the Board passed judgement on the 'reasonability' of professional opinions voiced by some of the medical men:

> We cannot but observe that the inconvenience and privations to which the sick ... were subjected seem to have made an impression upon Dr. Morewood's mind out of all proportion to the degree in which they appear from the rest of the Evidence to have existed.[42]

And, further, that Dr Neale had 'been much deceived' regarding some of the matters he had put forward.[43] Ultimately, the Board found that everything that could have been done, had been done, and that the mortality rate 'seems to be about that which should have been expected'.[44]

The concerns raised by Neale, Tice and their fellow medical officers were based on issues of hospital administration and the method of provisioning care to the soldiers housed in those hospitals. As such, they fell into the broadly sanitary part of the military medical remit – the part over which military officers traditionally had some supervisory role. However, the complaints they made were extremely serious and the non-inclusion of a medically trained expert on the investigating board demonstrates the degree to which the military felt it was competent to decide on the propriety of such matters, and also that military medical officers were willing to submit to that control. Indeed, a medical officer, Knight, had requested it. However, there is some indication that the military command would have preferred these matters to be handled within the medical department; as noted previously Pepys and Keate were censured severely for their decision to bring the matter forward.[45] The complaints voiced by Tice and Neale were, no doubt, motivated primarily by their concerns for the sick. However, in the context of the debate over regimental and general hospitals, and the well-known tensions within the Board, their complaints must also be seen as an attempt to curry favour with their chosen patrons. McGrigor's practical response to the problem, and his loyal support of the army and its medical department, stand in stark contrast to Neale's un-military approach, which it appears may have jeopardized his future with the AMD. Later in the Wars, it was rumoured that Neale had been 'blacklisted' for promotion by Wellington, on account of his book about his service in 1808–9, and the criticisms made therein about the army and its medical arrangements.[46]

McGrigor's canny incorporation of military norms in his approach to medicine, and in his relations with others in the medical department, also separates him from his predecessor in the Peninsula, Dr James Franck, and may account, in part, for the inability of the latter to succeed in the role.

James Franck, 1809–11

The Peninsular campaigns of Sir Arthur Wellesley began in April 1809, when he returned to Portugal. As described in Chapter 2, it was soon after this, in January 1810, that the old AMB was disbanded and a new Board, with Sir John Weir at its head, established. The new AMB was significantly more involved in the supervision of its leading medical officers, and also in directing the activities and medical investigations of army medical officers generally. Blanco states that its members 'plagued their inspectors in the field with directives and admonitions ... [displaying] a zeal for strict accounting of medical supplies'.[47] While this assessment of the new AMB is broadly accurate, it is important to consider also how interventionist the it was in medical matters, and what effects that had on the administration of medical services in the Peninsula.

Dr James Franck had replaced Dr Shapter as inspector of hospitals in the Peninsula and, accordingly, was at the head of the medical department of Wellesley's army. Franck was a Cambridge man and Cantlie describes him as 'very distinguished', but very little is known about him. His ability to integrate himself within military networks is called into question, both by his actions in the Peninsula and (as will be recalled from Chapter 3) his replacement by Dr Thomas Young at the head of the medical service in Egypt at Abercrombie's insistence. The army in the Peninsula presented its medical department with significant challenges as it campaigned up and down the country, particularly in the area of medical evacuation and the movement of sick and wounded from regimental hospitals to general hospitals in the rear.[48] Franck has been labelled by most commentators as an advocate of general hospitals. However, it is entirely probable that he saw no alternative for his charges, given the restrictions placed by Wellington on the conveyance of the sick and wounded with the army, because of a shortage of wagons and carts. To understand the scope of Franck's task, it is necessary to provide a short overview of the military campaigns that were undertaken during his tenure in the Peninsula.

After arriving in Portugal, Wellesley lost no time attacking the French forces under General Soult at Oporto in May 1809 and followed that success in the south at Talavera on 28 July. Despite appalling casualties,[49] he was victorious, and was made Viscount Wellington. The battle has been notable in medical histories for the heroic surgical efforts of George Guthrie, who was acting in charge of the medical arrangements because Franck had been struck down with dysentery.[50] The situation of the men wounded at the battle was rendered even more desperate because Wellington was unable to linger in the area after reports came to him of a French threat to the British line of communications, forcing him to move swiftly on to Oropesa. Many of the wounded were left to the mercies of the enemy, while others chose to literally drag themselves to the general hospital at Truxillo. In August, Wellington withdrew his entire army to the fortress of Badajoz, the area of which was unfortunately rife with malaria. Cantlie states that by 1 November, 9,016 men were in hospital.[51] In the hope of improving the health of the men, Wellington moved the bulk of the army north to the area east of Coimbra in December and the troops went into winter quarters.

In May 1810, the next campaign opened when Marshal Ney attacked the fortress of Cuidad Rodrigo, which fell six weeks later, closely followed by the fall of Almeida. Wellington's army had been reinforced over the winter period, but unfortunately many of the reinforcements were men who had served at Walcheren, and who suffered from recurring bouts of sickness throughout the course of the Peninsular War. At this time Wellington also had the command of a new Portuguese army, trained by General William Carr Beresford. The British forces retreated in the face of Ney's advance, but made a stand at Busaco on 27 September, where the majority of wounded were treated in the regimental hospitals and the severely wounded sent to the general hospital at Coimbra. Thereafter the army retreated to Lisbon where it sat untouchable behind the formidable lines of Torres Vedras. The wounded were transported from Coimbra to Lisbon and the majority of the sick were accommodated in the general hospitals there. Over the next few months, those hospitals became very crowded as the army suffered through the malarial season, and an increase in typhus over the winter.

In March 1811, the French army, which had camped opposite the lines, decamped and retreated towards Spain. The British pursued them. Meanwhile, in the south of the country, the force left behind under Beresford had engaged in several battles, culminating in a terrible confrontation at Albuera in May. George Guthrie had been serving with that army, and once again distinguished himself working for several days without rest operating on the wounded.[52]

It is apparent that Wellington was conscious of the needs of the medical department and did what he could to ensure it received the resources it required, particularly in requesting additional hospital mates to support the duties carried out at the general hospitals. His letters also reveal his concern at the depletion of regimental medical staff who were being used up by the general hospitals and thereby jeopardizing the health of soldiers on campaign.[53] Wellington also issued general orders giving military support to his medical officers, ensuring that soldiers who did not comply with their treatment regimes were to be reported to their commanding officers,[54] and enforcing cleanliness and hygiene.[55] However, despite Wellington's support in these matters, Dr Franck was unhappy with the position of the medical department in the army.

The AMB's correspondence with Franck reveals that Franck was dissatisfied with the respect accorded to his position:

> We entirely agree with you that the Chief Medical Officer in a situation similar to the one you now hold should be better paid, and that he should have the word 'General' restored ... We think however that the smallness of Pay or want of the Title alluded to should not be the means of producing degradation ... But it would be satisfactory to us that you look on occasion of pointing out the particulars in which you have found yourself and the Department degraded in Lord Wellington's Army[56]

It also appears that Franck may have actively participated in movements of discontent amongst the medical officers, in one letter the AMB make reference to rumours that there was considerable dissatisfaction among the medical officers, and that, 'we even understood that letters had been written by an officer of respectable rank adverting to your participation in the discontent.'[57]

At this time, Franck was struggling with problems in the general hospitals, such as the employment of soldiers as servants by the medical officers, and inconstant attendance at the hospitals by medical officers, both of which unfortunately merited the attention of Wellington who forbade the practice in his general orders.[58] The employment by medical officers of soldiers 'lingering' at the general hospitals was also expressly forbidden, on pain of court martial.[59] Not surprisingly, the AMB were alarmed by the appearance of these orders and requested that Franck would provide more detail on the transgressions. However, Franck appears to have been extremely sensitive to suggestions of criticism from the AMB, and took severe umbrage at this and later requests for information. Franck's failure to inform the Board of these matters, and the responses given by himself and his deputy, Inspector Bolton, suggest that not only were they hypersensitive, but they both deeply resented the incursion into, and oversight of, their practice by the AMB. A suggestion of the tenor of Franck's response is provided in the following letter from the AMB:

> You cannot surely, seriously believe that in requesting you to inform us of the grounds of Lord Wellington's order directing the medical officers to be always in the wards of the Hospital we could have had any ultimate view of such an improper and unmilitary measure as that of asking it, either by ourselves, or through you, of his Lordship! And in thus barely mentioning the subject again to you, we have only to express our regret that there should be any source whatever of irritation in your mind capable of influencing you to propose such a measure to us.[60]

It seems that Franck was so incensed by some of the AMB's criticisms that he wrote advising it on the ways in which it should behave, and what material it should take into account, prompting a very clear response from the AMB that it was in charge, not him.[61] In all their responses the new AMB were quick to point out the 'unmilitariness' of Franck's behaviour and suggestions, in contrast to their own. The new Board also enforced this concept in their dealings with other senior medical officers, on several occasions writing to Dr Borland in Sicily about insubordinate conduct in other doctors he had complained of and expressing the hope that those doctors would, in future 'conduct himself according to the rules of the service',[62] adding that Borland must himself comply with military conventions in disciplining those men, and involve the commander of the forces in such business.[63] Indeed, the expectation of medical officers to conduct themselves in 'military' fashion extended even to how they were to express their disapproval of the medical practice of medical officers placed above them. The court-martial of Surgeon Bash established that it was behaviour 'unbecoming an officer', to write to either the inspector of hospitals, or the head of the AMD at home, concerning the character of another medical officer without the knowledge and consent of the commanding officer.[64]

The requirement of 'military' behaviour was clearly difficult for some senior medical officers who were used to a great deal of autonomy in their practice. However, the new AMB's involvement in the actual medical practices of its officers was an even greater step away from the way the department had operated in the past. The AMB was extremely blunt in a directive sent to both Franck and Sir James Fellowes (heading the medical department at Cadiz) regarding its disapproval of the number of invalids being sent home. It was critical both of the number:

> Should the General in Command direct that the sick be indiscriminately sent home
> of course these distresses are not to be avoided, but otherwise we recommend to you
> to appoint a Board of Medical Officers for the purposes of examining the Patients in
> Hospital and of selecting the cases it may be proper to send to England[65]

and of the negligence it perceived in the arrangements: 'it may be fairly presumed that so great a number would not have perished had they remained at Lisbon, or at all events they would not have died under the miserable circumstances which must necessarily be the case at sea'.[66] It was also very specific about the matters that should be taken into consideration in the medical assessment of invalids proposed for return, including their likely recovery, the season at which they were proposed to be transported, and the records that should be kept by medical officers accompanying those who were sent home.[67] Despite Franck's protestations about this letter the AMB were not to be swayed, even subtly calling into question the medical judgement that had originally prompted the return home of the invalids:

> Our observations were meant to be general, not personal, nor do we see any thing,
> notwithstanding what you have said, for changing the sentiments that gave rise to

the letter in question: our opinion generally is that no men whatever should be sent home, upon the *abstract belief* that the climate of England would be more favourable to their recovery than the spot of service. It is the duty of medical officers employed to select invalids, to take also into consideration the circumstances to which they must be exposed in passing from one country to another, which officers of *sufficient military medical experience* must know are sufficient to counteract any benefit that might result from the climate they are to be sent to[68]

A similar guiding hand can be ascertained in the AMB's directions to Sir James Fellowes to investigate a fever prevalent in Cadiz at this time. The AMB acknowledged the relevance of Fellowes's local knowledge, but stated that as the fever was a contagion, 'some of the Laws of which being understood' it did not expect the fever should occasion too much mortality and gave him specific advice about the separation of the sick troops from the rest. He was also given directions to produce detailed reports on the progress, and nature of the disease.[69] In a further letter, the Board referred to the desirability of ascertaining whether the fever was similar to that which had appeared in Gibraltar in 1804, or to the yellow fever of the West Indies, and proceeded to lecture Fellowes on the appearances of yellow fever, and on how he might proceed to investigate the question; no doubt, all information already possessed by the distinguished doctor.[70]

Despite its best efforts, the AMB was unable to secure the medical staff required by Franck in the Peninsula, sending him instead hospital mates of a lower standard than they had considered doing before, who were 'equal only to the lowest offices in the department'.[71] These men of 'slender qualifications' were designated 'warrant mates' and prohibited from promotion without further education in the 'regular schools at home'.

The most interesting aspect of the letters from the AMB to Franck, however, is the indication that Franck experienced a fraught relationship with Wellington. The AMB was pained to observe:

> though with some reluctance, as it is a point of great delicacy ... that 'you scarcely know how to request Lord Wellington to put his signature to so many papers'. This as well as other parts of your communications seem to bespeak feelings, for which we trust there is no solid foundation[72]

Franck was advised to forward the bulk of the materials through Wellington's secretary. Despite this advice, however, it seems that he was still unwilling to discuss the medical arrangements of the army with Wellington:

> With respect to what you say about not wishing to give trouble to Lord Wellington we have only to refer you to what is mentioned in one of our former letters, on a similar occasion; the necessary business of the Army must be done, let it occasion trouble to whom it may.[73]

However, the AMB chose to accept letters from Wellington conveying his approbation of the work of the medical officers in the Peninsula, as proof that all was well.[74] Despite this, the fact that Wellington felt compelled to write such letters, and the existence of newspaper reports and rumours to which the AMB also adverted in the same letter, indicate that all was certainly not well. Franck left the service in the summer of 1811, invalided to England for health reasons. An unfortunately enduring portrait was painted of him by Guthrie, who encountered him sitting at the side of the road apparently confused and out of his depth on the way to the Coa River in September that year. Alluding to Franck's 'unmilitary' character, Guthrie stated that 'he was one of the best men in the world, but having slept out all night, looked as unhappy as need be for a man not used to it, and not a little frightened withal'.[75] However, Franck had not finished with the AMD and took all his official papers with him to England, where he made hard work of giving them back for McGrigor's use.[76] This was possibly an act of petulance, but it seems more likely that his retention of these papers was down to his inability to see his practice as part of an overarching military machine, or as a statement of his resistance to the oversight of that practice.

Franck may not have been the success McGrigor was in the Peninsula, but his tenure is not irrelevant to medical historians. Through his difficult relationship with Wellington, and his disputes with the AMB, a picture of the growing militarization of the medical service begins to appear. A militarization that Franck failed to assimilate, and for which failing he was gently criticized by those who had, like Guthrie. The tendency of the AMB to try and supervise the medical practice of its leading officers was better resisted by McGrigor, who employed his skills in recruiting military officers to help him maintain medical independence. The complicated manoeuvring that was required in an army where military officers felt competent to assess the management of hospitals, and where increasing attempts were made to establish standard medical practices, was something that could only successfully be negotiated by those who embraced military medicine as a substantially different practice to civilian medicine.

The Portuguese Service

In early 1809, General William Carr Beresford was placed in command of the Portuguese army and British officers were attached to all the newly formed Portuguese units. Beresford's achievement in creating an efficient fighting force in a short space of time was praised highly by Wellington and has drawn the admiration of military historians. A similar transformation was performed on the medical service by William Fergusson, who was appointed inspector general of hospitals to the Portuguese army.[77] However, the work of Fergusson and the British medical officers who served with the Portuguese army has never properly been investigated.[78] This section will set out the problems faced by Fergusson in that role, and demonstrate how his response, and that of the medical officers under him, provides evidence of a strong and united medical philosophy developing among military medical officers at this time and a growing sophistication in the ways in which military and medical officers were interacting. Fergusson's ongoing promotion of military medicine as a specialty will also be considered.

Fergusson had been educated at the Academy at Ayr (his hometown), and had taken his MD at the University in Edinburgh, afterwards serving an apprenticeship in Edinburgh and walking the wards in London. He entered the army in 1794 as an assistant surgeon, and had served in the Low Countries, St Domingo, the Baltic and Britain before proceeding to the Peninsula where he acted as principal medical officer between Shapter's departure and Franck's arrival.[79] He wrote an account of his medical career late in his life, and his official papers from the Wars also survive.[80] From these documents, a detailed account of his work in the Portuguese army can be compiled.

Fergusson was not reluctant to engage in disputes with his medical colleagues, and was particularly sensitive to any suggestion of 'insubordination' from those beneath him. While deputy inspector of hospitals in England, he brought a regimental surgeon to a general court martial, for neglect of his duty and 'for disregarding [Fergusson's] orders to improve his work'.[81] Throughout the rest of his career, he exhibited the same high expectations of his staff, and a distinctly militaristic approach to reprimanding medical officers who fell short of them. He was a fervent advocate of regimental hospitals which he called the 'cardinal hinge on which the health of armies depends'[82] and, like McGrigor, won the favour of Francis Knight.[83] The debate over regimental and general hospitals was far from over at the start of the Peninsular War. Some officers, like Alexander Lessassier pursued careers in the general hospitals for personal comfort and to make professional connections.[84] Others like Adam Neale advocated general hospitals as essential to the health of the army.[85] However, an incident that occurred before Fergusson entered the Portuguese service, suggests that support for the regimental system was becoming very widespread amongst the medical staff of the army.

Around June 1809, when Fergusson was acting head of the medical department with Wellesley's army, he engaged in a dispute with an older practitioner, Dr Thomas Ross.[86] Fergusson had criticized Ross's work, prompting Ross to write to Wellesley complaining of Fergusson's conduct. Most importantly, Ross represented Fergusson's criticism to be motivated by a significant difference in medical philosophy:

> [Fergusson] very naturally wishes to get rid of an officer older and more experienced in the service, than himself, and one who disapproves most decidedly of the late attempts made by the Inspectorial Department to practice the reveries of Dr. Jackson

... and to manage the sick and wounded soldiers of an Army on Service without a regular establishment of General Hospitals.[87]

Ross's attribution of the regimental system to Robert Jackson indicates that although Jackson was, at this time, *persona non grata* with the AMD, his influence and reputation were wide-ranging.[88]

Fergusson had an extremely strong reaction to Ross's allegations and sent a circular letter to all the principal medical officers superintending brigades with the army saying that he had been accused 'from vile motives and by the adoption of a bad system [to have] deprived the sick of the comforts and protection they are entitled to'. He asked them to consult with all the medical officers in their brigades and send an answer giving their opinion of whether the sick of the army had been well cared for.[89] He was particular in asking them to consult widely amongst their staff, as he wanted to give Wellesley the 'fullest information'. This extraordinary appeal produced a flurry of replies from the senior medical officers of the army, who all wrote to say that they were in full support of, and agreement with, Fergusson.[90] Even if we make some allowance for the probability that some medical officers were likely to have decided to support their commanding officer over an ageing staff surgeon, these responses indicate that a belief in the benefits of using the regimental system in armies had become widespread amongst the medical officers in the British army by this time. It appears that Ross came out of the affair badly, and was prohibited by Wellesley from serving as a staff surgeon in Portugal.[91]

While this dispute was in progress, Wellesley had written to the commander-in-chief asking that deputy inspector of hospitals, Thompson, be replaced at the head of the Portuguese medical service, because Wellesley, who had past experience with that gentlemen, believed him to be too old and not equal to the duties of the situation. Wellesley requested a more 'efficient' medical officer.[92] According to McGrigor, Beresford specifically requested that he be appointed to the post, but his appointment had to be cancelled when McGrigor was sent to Walcheren in October.[93] McGrigor stated that he was then 'mainly instrumental' in having Fergusson appointed in his stead.[94] In the meantime, a contingent of twelve medical officers appointed staff surgeons to the Portuguese army,[95] had proceeded to Portugal and, for want of a senior officer 'arrived ... under many disadvantages'.[96] However, one surgeon reported that even with this 'little band of British medical officers, Marshal Beresford was able, in a great measure, to stem the dreadful tide of mortality which, at one time, threatened to leave him without a soldier in the field'.[97]

British accounts of Portuguese medicine (in fact, all aspects of Portuguese life) were highly coloured by their belief in a superstitious, dirty and backward Portuguese national character – largely sourced in British prejudice against

Catholicism and Catholic ritual.[98] Dr Andrew Halliday commented that 'In Portugal the Physicians seem, in the practical part of their profession, to be about a century behind the rest of Europe'.[99] Similar sentiments were voiced by Schaumann, a commissary:

> Medicine, surgery and the treatment of illness are still in their infancy in this country, although the Portuguese doctors will not admit it ... I can testify to the fact that I have come across many doctors here who were quacks, and have, as a rule, found their surgical instruments obsolete, rusty, and few in number. They seem to know nothing about the latest discoveries.[100]

Assistant Surgeon Broughton thought the same, and commented on the antiquated education the Portuguese medical officers had received:

> Whenever I met with medical men I uniformly found their science limited to a degree which almost exceeds belief. Their study is chiefly confined to the perusal of a few old authors, whose practice among us has become obsolete; and they have consequently few conceptions beyond the dogmas of the latter.[101]

The prevailing low opinion of Portuguese medicine was linked to the Portuguese abhorrence of the lancet and refusal to use mercury in the treatment of venereal disease. However, as will be shown, British observation of some Portuguese practices led military medical officers to challenge some received medical learning in the years after the Wars.

When he arrived in early 1810, Fergusson's task was Herculean. The Portuguese medical department was run by a central Junta in Lisbon, comprising the physician-general of the army, the surgeon general, and the contador-fiscal. According to Halliday, these, and other senior appointments within the service, were 'complete sinecures' and their duties were performed by assistants with little experience. He also alleged that the general and regimental staff performed very little duty, making no appearance at their brigades and only slightly more at the general hospitals, that in fact 'they had retired to remote quarters of the kingdom, and there lived in idleness, enjoying the fruits of their pensions, or pursuing private practice'.[102] The traditional division between physic and surgery was rigorously enforced: surgeons of the regiments were prohibited from working on medical cases and also from encroaching on the territory of the apothecaries by compounding or mixing drugs. Although surgeons were permitted to perform operations and dress wounds, supplies of the necessary implements prevented them from doing so, and most sick soldiers ended up in the general hospitals from whence they almost never returned to their corps.[103]

At the general hospitals Halliday said that 'civil Physicians, combined with the local departments, and supported by the government, reaped *their* full harvest of sinecure and peculation'.[104] Another advocate of the regimental system,

Halliday argued that the Portuguese soldiers, once fallen into the 'traps' of the general hospitals were impossible to remove, even when restored to health.[105] Furthermore, the general hospitals were 'a den of thieves', where there was no shadow of discipline, 'and the picture which most of the general hospitals exhibited may be conceived, but cannot possibly be described'.[106]

One of the first British contingent of medical officers to the Portuguese service, Staff Surgeon Thomas, who arrived before Fergusson's appointment, reported to Thomas Keate his first impressions of the Portuguese medical service, attributing many of its problems to the fact that the physicians and surgeons of the general hospitals were not under military control: 'the whole concern is so badly ordered and so little calculated for military purposes ... I have very strongly recommended that the sick should be taken care of Regimentally'.[107] He also noted, in closing, that he had not been provided with any medicine or surgical instruments, and that he believed all the other British medical officers were in the same situation.

Upon Fergusson's arrival, it appears that he sent a letter to all the staff surgeons, requesting information about their stations, and setting out his proposed changes to the service. Those reforms centred on the implementation of a regimental hospital system and the extension of the regimental plan to general hospitals. The responses he received were unanimous in supporting his proposal to establish a system on the British regimental plan.[108] He was usually counselled that the system in place would be easier to just sweep aside, than to improve. Some of the impetus for the establishment of regimental hospitals may have originated in the inability of the British staff surgeons to exert any authority in the Portuguese general hospitals, where affronted native practitioners ignored them.[109] Assertions of the ability of military medical officers to provide both medical and surgical care can also be found in these responses, possibly articulated because of the purely surgical role into which the Portuguese tried to relegate the British.[110] The most common criticisms voiced of the Portuguese system were the lack of military control in the hospitals, their general filthiness and the lack of necessary supplies. Surgeon Jebb wrote 'I know of nothing that would prove more useful than a supply of mops and scrubbing brushes'.[111]

Fergusson and his staff surgeons diligently set about implementing their regimental plan. However, they encountered resistance from the Portuguese in doing this, prompting Fergusson to write:

> Will you have the goodness to submit the enclosed letter from Dr. Halliday to the Marshal, with my request, that he would be pleased to signify in general orders his approbation of the sick, being treated in regimental or Brigade Hospitals whenever it is practicable. The Portuguese have no conception of what these hospitals mean, and resist everything that is new.[112]

Fergusson also stated in that letter that the Physico Mor of the Portuguese army (the physician general), had been actively de-establishing regimental hospitals 'as soon as my back was turned'. Fergusson had some success convincing the Portuguese to change their ways, after writing a 'kind of manifesto to the native Doctors of my intentions' that he said 'electrified the Medicos of Coimbra where the Hospitals are now perfect and beautiful'.[113] However, he was soon to become embroiled in a bitter feud with the physician general and by June they were both in a 'confounded rage'.[114] The dispute appears to have followed Fergusson's manifesto and probably related to their competing ideas about the proper way to run the medical department, and their disagreement over which one of them was in charge. The matter degenerated when Fergusson took offence at some comments made by Staff Surgeon Robertson (who had defended the physician general) about Fergusson's reforms, and also about Staff Surgeon Halliday. Fergusson got into such a fury that he wrote to Beresford demanding Robertson be charged with 'scandalous and infamous conduct in calumniating and defaming his superior officer', Robertson having had the temerity to suggest that Fergusson's reforms were nothing new, and had already been anticipated by Beresford's orders.[115] Fergusson also wrote to Weir,[116] and to Brigadier General Blunt who was in charge of the recruitment depot in Peniche.[117] While Blunt was very sympathetic, Beresford was less so. Beresford and Wellington criticized Fergusson for drawing Blunt into the matter, and agreed that the matter had better not be brought forward. Beresford also defended Robertson's statements about Halliday, expressing the opinion that he had probably just passed on rumours he had actually heard, reminding Fergusson that there was 'among the Portuguese Medical Men a party against Mr. Halliday'.[118]

Blunt was in charge of the recruitment depot at Peniche and wrote to Fergusson several times over the latter part of 1810 begging him to make an attendance there.[119] Blunt reported that the men were dying in droves and was 'apprehensive that it is a great want of talent' causing the deaths. His letters reveal his extreme frustration at not being able to do anything about it, or obtain help he considered competent. His letters to Fergusson reveal a personal friendship and a great respect for his professional abilities. It appears that Fergusson was not permitted to make the journey, and after making requests for help for over three months, Blunt was not shy in voicing his disgust with the Portuguese government, who could let so many die.[120] Fergusson was also appalled at the mortality at Peniche, and following year, he took pains to ensure that the recruitment depot was located at Mafra, in the healthier mountainous region.[121] Fergusson later cited this incident in his memoir as evidence that military officers should pay more heed to their medical advisors.[122]

It does not seem that Fergusson's position markedly improved over the next year. In mid-1811, Fergusson approached Franck stating that the Portuguese refused to give him any duties and that he possessed 'not even the shadow of authority'. He petitioned Franck to take the matter before Wellington, suggesting that it was impossible to achieve anything as long as the Portuguese practitioners were not amenable to martial law and were so miserably paid.[123] This may not have been the only representation made to Wellington about the Portuguese army; in December he issued the following General Order:

> The Commander of the Forces has received frequent complaints from Officers, as well of the Portuguese as of the British army, belonging to the civil as well as the military departments, of the uncivil, and, in various instances, insulting language, in which some of the communications in writing are carried on. It is impossible that the service should not suffer, if those who are to assist each other do not agree; and it cannot be expected that they should agree, if harsh, uncivil, and insulting terms are used in their necessary communications.[124]

In June 1811, the physician general informed Fergusson that he had no authority or position in the Portuguese army.[125] Fergusson was alarmed, and attempted to resolve the problem with a new plan for the regulation of the medical department. He presented it to Beresford on 14 July 1811.[126] In it, he focused on the importance of the regimental hospital to the health of the army, but he also stressed the importance of having experienced medical officers 'of good education who have acquired experience of Military practice, with a knowledge of the Soldier, his diseases, temper and habits in Regimental Hospitals', implicitly degrading the possible contribution of the Portuguese practitioners. Accordingly, his plan also put him in charge of all the military hospitals of the Kingdom, while the physician general would live in Lisbon and regulate only appointments and supplies. Importantly, Fergusson also suggested that all hospitals should be considered military establishments and all persons employed in them subject to martial law.

Fergusson and his staff surgeons continued to have problems with authority and medical supplies, and Fergusson suffered slights from the Portuguese who decided not to recognize his rank in the allocation of billeted accommodation.[127] The extensive use of civilian practitioners by the Portuguese was not halted. Fergusson wrote of his inspection of a Portuguese hospital at Viseu, where he found 'the low state of wretchedness which ever characterizes Portuguese management, when ever their miserable beings are committed to the care of civil practitioners'.[128] He was not alone in this opinion. Surgeon John Griffith wrote at this time that he was disgusted with the manner of carrying on Portuguese duty.[129] Frictions were also being expressed over the diagnosis and treatment of men at the depot of recruits at Mafra, where British medical officers had reported an epidemic of scurvy, but the physician sent to investigate by the Portuguese government diagnosed only a local infection of the teeth and gums.[130] Fergusson investigated at the depot and wrote to Beresford that the disease was, in fact, the true scurvy. In his letter he carefully set out the causes of the disease, explaining that the Portuguese physicians did not have the requisite experience to diagnose the disease at the early stage in which it was presenting. Perhaps hoping to appeal to military sensibilities, he pointed to the damaging effects of the disease on the efficacy of the Royal British Navy prior to the discovery that 'acid fruits' could cure it, and was quick to state that General Blunt had by that means arrested the disease.[131]

It was at about this time that Andrew Halliday escalated divisions between the British and Portuguese establishments. His *Observations of the Present State of the Portuguese Army* was dedicated to Beresford, and was almost certainly intended to praise the Marshal's efforts. However, Halliday's tactless descriptions of the Portuguese, their army, and especially their medical department, resulted in his being thrown out of the Portuguese service.[132] Wellington stated that he could not 'consent to any officer remaining in the Country who has rendered himself so obnoxious to its Government'.[133] The book was not well received by some of his staff surgeon colleagues who branded him 'a Judas among the doctors attached to the Portuguese army'.[134] But others very much regretted his dismissal.[135] Halliday himself apparently reported only that he had 'been removed *not exactly* in the way that he wished'.[136] Indeed, the Portuguese service which had initially been very attractive to many British medical officers no longer had much appeal, some even turned down appointments on the grounds that 'although it gives more pay it is not pleasant nor comfortable'.[137] Not surprisingly, by March of 1812, Fergusson was heartily sick of his situation with the Portuguese and was endeavouring, unsuccessfully, to get out.[138]

Over the next few months, staff surgeons continued to complain of disputes with the 'native' practitioners, and of a want of authority to make the necessary changes in their hospitals or to enforce treatments. Military officers were also keen to get their men out of the general hospitals and into regimental establishments.[139] Despite the obstacles of Portuguese resistance and obtaining supplies, there were gradual improvements in this direction. However, Fergusson was exasperated with the Portuguese physicians, and in his investigation of excessive mortality at the depot in Mafra made the serious accusation that 'much of the fatality may be justly ascribed to the malpractice of the Physicians'.[140] He went on to try and convince Blunt of his medical opinion not with what he called 'professional talk' but with the 'language of common sense' denouncing the physicians' failure to procure evacuations or to use bloodletting with agricultural analogies. He finally stated:

> I think further that these prejudices may justly be attributed to them as crimes as they
> for the most part obstinately refuse to be instructed even by the example of death or
> to communicate on the subject with the British Medical Officers, the comparison of
> whose practice with their own as founded on greater experience of Military diseases
> would in all probability dissipate errors to which they are so much attracted.[141]

After making these strong observations, Fergusson requested Blunt to make the treatment of the sick the subject of a military regulation.

Not long after, Fergusson received intelligence from Staff Surgeon William Wynn that 'the patron' (Beresford) had agreed and settled a new plan for the government of hospitals with the secretary at war. This new plan would make Fergusson 'co-equal' with the physician general in all respects. Under the plan the physician general would remain in Lisbon, and Fergusson would be attached to headquarters in the field. Beresford apparently hoped that this plan would end his 'plague with the hospitals'.[142] He also intended to place a general officer over both the physician general and Fergusson, and 'would have permanent Governors of hospitals'. Beresford must have submitted his new 'Regulamento' to Fergusson for his comments. In November 1812, Fergusson wrote criticizing the proposal, stating that the physician general was only a 'physician from civil life' while he was a 'military medical officer, having passed his life in the service'. He argued that the British had been appointed to the Portuguese service to give its medical officers the benefit of their military experience and rejected the proposed position of surgeon general because it would not allow him to direct those civilian practitioners in military practice, and would be inferior in rank to the physician general. He also perceived that it would restrict him to communicating with the government on matters of surgery. Instead Fergusson suggested an alternative model, which gave him more authority based on his military experience. Importantly, he argued that Beresford's plan would make Portuguese physicians always superior to British medical officers, but that those British medical officers were not 'surgeons alone, but medical officers, medically educated to perform Military Medical Duties'. He concluded by stating his resentment at being treated thus far as someone who had just come to 'sweep and clean', and asserting his desire not to be placed in 'in a situation to be slighted and despised by a village doctor of Portugal'.[143]

Two weeks after sending this memorandum to Beresford, Fergusson was ordered to the side of McGrigor and left the Portuguese service.[144] His time with the Portuguese service was undoubtedly one beset with difficulties and obstacles, in dealing with which he may not have had the unreserved support of his commander-in-chief. Fergusson's failure to recruit Beresford to his cause was most likely the result of his stiff and unbending character that could not, or would not, pursue efficiency over personal slights. However, Fergusson's commitment to the regimental plan and his use of military systems to enforce medical doctrine was reflected (more successfully) in the strategies employed by McGrigor. In the final months of his service with the Portuguese, Fergusson's attempts to win military officers over display an intriguing adaptation of medical language and thought to what he perceived would be familiar and readily understood concepts to military minds.[145] Most military officers appear to have been supportive of the efforts of the medical officers in Portugal and endorsed the regimental model they were striving to implement. Equally, medical officers repeatedly emphasized to their military patrons that their practice of 'military medicine' was special, and that unlike the Portuguese doctors, they were a part of the army, and subject to martial rule – a point that was particularly stressed as being integral to the provision of an efficient service, but also one that limited the autonomy of the practitioner. The determined resistance all British medical officers encountered in their dealings with the 'native' doctors sharpened their sense of what it was that made them special, and as Fergusson suggested, more than just 'surgeons alone'.

Conclusion

Many of the issues that captured the attention of army medical practitioners during the first half of the Peninsular War were those that had been debated during previous campaigns: the relative merits of regimental and general hospitals; the extent to which they should operate independently; and the importance of on-the-field training for military medical practice. However, the environment in which military medical officers were operating had changed with the appointment of a new and more interventionist AMB, and the increasing interest of military officers in the operations of the department. Successful practitioners responded to these pressures by embracing military culture, not only personally but also in the practice of their medicine. By doing so, they were able to achieve the dual objectives of securing a more independent practice, and further endorsing the idea that they were substantially distinct from their civilian counterparts. The practitioner who best embodied and promoted all the aspects of this militarization in the Peninsula was McGrigor, and his impact on the medical department there is discussed in the following chapter.

5 JAMES MCGRIGOR IN THE PENINSULA

Throughout the preceding chapters, McGrigor has frequently been identified as an important figure in the militarization of army medicine and in the promotion of the military medical officer identity. His appointment as inspector of hospitals in the Peninsula, and his subsequent role at the head of the AMD made him arguably the most influential individual in military medicine during, and for the half century following, the Peninsular War. This chapter will focus on McGrigor in the Peninsula, and will reconsider the traditional account of his time there in the context of the conclusions about military medicine already advanced. It will go on to discuss how and why McGrigor cultivated the patronage of Wellington, and the importance of that process to the military medical officer identity and to the militarization of army medicine.

The official writings, publications, records and personal letters of such an important figure should be subject to rigorous examination, but McGrigor's autobiography (which lingers on his time in the Peninsula) has been adopted almost without question by his biographer, Blanco, and other historians of the Wars such as Cantlie. These narratives are traditionally dominated by accounts of his 'warm relationship' with Wellington, his administrative reforms in the general hospitals and in casualty evacuation, and his innovations in medical returns. McGrigor is also credited with significant achievements in the elevation of the status of medical officers. Together, these form an oft-repeated triumphal medical history of the final years of the Wars. In concert with the surgical innovations and successes of the other 'hero' of the theatre, George Guthrie, the picture presented by most historians is one of improvement and success (although tempered by the failures which McGrigor also bewailed, the inability of the army to provide adequate means for the transport of the wounded and the scarcity of properly educated medical staff). McGrigor's success in lowering mortality rates by the winter of 1812–13 has been identified by Napier as contributing the equivalent of an extra division to the army at the battle of Vitoria, and by Blanco as evidence that the medical department was central to Wellington's military machine.[1]

It is undeniable that during McGrigor's tenure, and largely because of his reforms, significant improvements were achieved by the AMD in the lowering of mortality, prevention of disease, efficiency of hospitals, the line of evacuation, production of returns and, to some extent, the status of medical officers. It is not intended that this chapter will contradict any of those claims, although it will examine more critically the nature of McGrigor's relationship with Wellington, especially in the context of McGrigor's relationship with the AMB.

The only history that has given more thoughtful consideration to McGrigor, the recent *Advancing with the Army*, is limited in its treatment of him owing to its focus on the education and progress of its 'cohort' as a body, using McGrigor only to illustrate certain points revealed by that research. Blanco's work does go further than previous treatments of the subject and embellishes the narrative provided in the autobiography with extracts from some official letters and summaries of the most important regulations issued by him in the Peninsula. Blanco also considers evidence of McGrigor's disagreements with the AMB and concludes that his correspondence is indicative of a man 'confident of Wellington's support'.[2] Despite this, Blanco does not consider the issues underlying those disagreements, the ways in which McGrigor enlisted Wellington, or the impact of his approach to these matters on other military medical officers, or on army medicine.

In this chapter that analysis will be undertaken; it will demonstrate how McGrigor's dealings with the new AMB affected his relationship with Wellington, and how his efforts to recruit Wellington to his cause contributed to the further militarization of army medicine and promotion of the military medical identity. McGrigor's self-appointed role as a medical 'hub' and his desire to standardize medical practice were refined and expanded in the Peninsula and this aspect of his administration will also be discussed. The writings of other practitioners will also be addressed in an effort to determine themes in the culture of military medical officers by this stage of the Wars.

Background to the Peninsula

Before considering McGrigor's activities in the Peninsula, it is necessary to trace briefly the development of his approach to military medicine while on service in Britain after the Egyptian campaign. Prior to his appointment in the Peninsula, McGrigor had served as the deputy inspector of the Northern District and then as the deputy inspector of the South West District in England. It was in the latter role, as discussed above, that he so admirably handled the crisis following the return of the sick from Corunna. In his correspondence from this time, his characteristic method of collating, refining, and disseminating the results of medical experiments and treatments is evident, as is his much commented upon penchant for accurate and timely returns from his staff. Importantly, this correspondence also demonstrates that, like Fergusson, McGrigor had embraced military structures and sanctions as one way of controlling the practice of his underlings. He too had a distinct lack of tolerance for 'insubordination', and wrote in 1805 of his nearly reporting a surgeon for the offence, but then relenting as the surgeon was 'new to orders'[3] (a letter which also shows that not all medical officers quickly accepted the military restrictions on the independence of practice and comment they exercised in civil life). However, it was not only in his direct dealings with subordinates that McGrigor was able to benefit from such military strictures. Similar techniques were used by his patron, Francis Knight, to ensure that junior officers who complained about McGrigor (and presumably other senior medical officers in Knight's favour) were brought into line. In one instance the complaints of a disgruntled junior officer precipitated the following use of intimidation by Knight, who wrote back:

> The Inspector General cannot but highly disapprove the unbecoming want of respect to your *superior officer* in which the language of your letter is couched, and if you mean to prefer a complaint against Mr McGrigor, Mr Knight expects you to transmit the same in a more precise form and order that Mr McGrigor may be officially called upon to repel the charge. The Inspector General will hope that you have duly furnished Deputy Inspector McGrigor, with the copy of a communication in which his name is — but lest you should not have done so, thro' inadvertence, the original has been transmitted to Beverly for his information.[4]

Military expectations were also useful in helping McGrigor to influence the medical practices of his staff. In 1806, he wrote to a junior surgeon that he was free to purchase certain therapeutics but cautioned him at the same time that it would 'not leave a good impression of his surgical skills' on the senior members of the AMB. McGrigor suggested to the hapless surgeon that weekly health inspections would serve him better in the future.[5] McGrigor promoted antiphlogistic therapies, particularly bloodletting in the treatment of pneumonia.[6] McGrigor also used his communications with military officers to advocate another of his favoured therapies, gestation (cure by travelling in open air, which had been much praised by Robert Jackson), stating to General Evelegh that it was a 'well known fact that motion and change of place frequently breaks the charm of disease whether contagious or not'.[7] By targeting military officers, as well as medical ones, regarding appropriate medical treatments McGrigor displayed a sophisticated understanding of the dual pathways necessary to ensure a welcome reception of his ideas within the military framework. It is unthinkable that McGrigor would have promoted regimes of treatment which he did not believe to be efficacious, but the treatments which he did favour had the distinctly military advantages of being inexpensive and not reliant on the provision of supplies. The roughness of heroic bleeding and exposure to the elements during a fever may also have had a distinctly robust, or Spartan, appeal to the military enthusiast.

However, despite his very meritorious service, his management of the Corunna disaster and Walcheren crisis, and his appeal to medical and military officers alike McGrigor did not escape the heavy hand of the new AMB. Although he appears to have had a generally good relationship with the new members, from October 1810 his correspondence books include many letters from the new AMB that either directly criticize his work, or suggest that he could have taken a better approach. The AMB expressed 'surprise' at his employment of 'so many medical attendants at Hilsea with such a ... small number of patients'.[8] It suggested his lack of organization had wasted time,[9] and made subtly negative comments about his medical reports, 'The Board ... do not understand how the faulty state of a Hospital can tend to produce disease though it may certainly retard the cure and induce relapses'.[10]

McGrigor's responses to these comments from the AMB were mild, expressing his 'exceeding regret' that his arrangements were not satisfactory to it, but also setting out in detail his case for how they had been appropriate for the situation.[11] Despite the lack of open defiance in his letters, the constant stream of criticism must have been a marked difference to the confidence he had experienced under Knight's patronage, and an increasing irritation to a professional man used to respect and autonomy. The AMB continued to address McGrigor in this fashion after his appointment to the head of the medical services in the Peninsula, and it was in that theatre that he began to resist and then to openly defy it. Blanco's assessment of McGrigor's defiant letters, as those of a man confident of Wellington's support, is accurate. However, what is more important is how McGrigor went about cultivating Wellington's support for his disputes with the AMB, and what impact that had on the conduct of medicine in the Peninsula.

McGrigor in the Peninsula – The Standard History

As has been stated, McGrigor's autobiography has been relied upon heavily in the production of medical histories of the Peninsular War. However, that work does not mention his difficulties with the AMB. Such issues will be discussed in the second half of this chapter, but first it is necessary to reconsider the 'standard' account. This section closely follows McGrigor's autobiography, and considers his motivations in writing it. It also sets that account within the context of the conclusions that have been reached about military medicine in the preceding chapters.

The story of McGrigor in the Peninsula usually relies on a standard sequence of 'scenes' between McGrigor and Wellington, which are drawn from the autobiography. These 'scenes' have achieved an almost mythic status in military medical histories of the period, and are said to establish the 'special relationship' between the two men. It appears that it was McGrigor's intention that the autobiography should represent him as being within the Duke's confidence and, as much as it was possible, as his friend. That relationship has been taken for granted by historians and cited as one of the principal reasons McGrigor was so successful in his medical reforms.

The usual account given of McGrigor's work in the Peninsula begins with his arrival in Portugal in January 1812 where he found the army sickly, its medical records in disarray and medical supplies badly organized. His first task was to address these problems, which he did very efficiently by completely reorganizing supply and accounting procedures. He then turned his attention to the glut of convalescing sick in Lisbon and the consequent concentration of medical officers at the same place. To disperse these men, he developed new guidelines for the movement of sick to the rear and the evacuation of deserving cases to Britain. He then made his way to Castello Bom to join Wellington and inspected the hospitals along his route. In each place he implemented his system of hospital organization, wherever possible having the sick separated by type of disease and degree of convalescence, and each group housed in separate wards and buildings. On this journey he also became very sensible of the horrors inflicted upon the sick and wounded as they were transported from one place to another in the notorious bullock carts of the country. When he arrived at headquarters he was gratified to find that Wellington recalled their previous meeting in India. His meeting with Wellington the following day provides the first 'scene' between the two men. It establishes McGrigor's mode of conducting business with the Duke and also informs the reader that McGrigor had daily one-on-one access to him. McGrigor conveys his sense that Wellington wanted a *military* medical officer, and that McGrigor fulfilled that requirement.

In this 'scene' McGrigor arrives at Wellington's office to give his report but is informed that he can leave the papers with the adjutant general. However, McGrigor stands his ground and states that Wellington had asked to see him personally. Wellington himself then appears at the door and calls McGrigor in. During the meeting, McGrigor quickly perceives that his written notes irritate Wellington – and in future, he always gives Wellington his report from memory. Wellington states during the interview that he wants an officer like McGrigor, who thoroughly understands the duties and habits of soldiers.[12] At that first meeting, McGrigor also puts to Wellington a plan for the improvement of the medical service to which Wellington agrees in as much as it relates to the prevention of malingering and the establishment of local medical boards, but not to the widespread adoption of regimental hospitals or the transport of wounded by spring wagons because he believes that those measures will impede the movements of his army.

McGrigor's commitment to getting the slight cases transported with the army, instead of being sent to the general hospitals, was one he pursued despite

Wellington's veto. Commanding officers of regiments wanted to do it, and in McGrigor's words soon the practice 'crept in'. Medical officers were also complicit in the plan, 'knowing [it] was one which I especially advocated, [they] entered readily into it'.[13] McGrigor's extraordinary disregard of Wellington's command has been passed over in existing histories. However, it provides an insight into his character and approach to the conduct of his duties. It demonstrates his determination to do what he believed was best and his skill in cultivating the support of military officers at all levels, not only those at the top, by providing a medical service that met their day-to-day needs as well as caring for the welfare of their men. It also shows that he was a risk-taker, and may be testament to his skills in reading the mind of his commander, as it is unlikely Wellington would have been unaware of the 'creeping' practice and must have tacitly supported it as long as it did not usher in the negative consequences he had predicted.

In March 1812, Wellington prepared to besiege Badajoz. In April, McGrigor was present at the height of Wellington's attempts to take the fort. The loss of life during the siege was terrible, and McGrigor used the 'scene' to emphasize his physical proximity to Wellington during and after the siege, and his place in Wellington's confidence by reporting his observation of Wellington's very private expression of grief after the victory. The siege is also notable for McGrigor's petitioning Wellington to acknowledge the efforts of the medical officers in his official report, which Wellington did, and which it has been argued was a significant step forward for the morale and status of military medical officers.[14]

McGrigor returned to headquarters at Freinada after the siege and in his autobiography records that nothing much occurred until the beginning of June. Blanco states that over those few months McGrigor extended his control over the medical department, issued regulations on the enforcement of hygienic standards in hospitals and established aid stations along routes from the line to the hospitals. He also made his expectations of good practice and extensive reporting clear to his officers. McGrigor's strong interest in the production of returns by medical officers has been much commented on by medical historians and his correspondence from this time does express frustration that the returns received were in an 'extremely incorrect state' and regretted 'the necessity of remitting some of them several times for correction'.[15] However, in the same letter to the AMB, he also stated that the returns he had received were often 'what is called "made up" conveying deception instead of information' and that he had made a change to the return which made it easier and less likely to lead to that practice. Despite his reputation for being fixated on returns, McGrigor defended his staff to the AMB during the resumption of the campaign season in August, stating that 'the professional duties of the Medical Officers do not allow them to make up [returns] at the present moment', and that his trial of the prescribed form demonstrated that it 'entails so much writing on the Medical Officers that I have given it up'. Furthermore, he reported that on the service it was the 'general remark' that 'the time of the medical officers is taken up in writing. I have dispensed with every return to myself which is not absolutely necessary: so as to enable the Medical Officer to devote his time to his patients.'[16]

Wellington's next campaign took him south into Castile, and to a great victory over the French at Salamanca in July. The movement of the army onward to Madrid provides the next, very important, 'scene' in the mythology of the Wellington–McGrigor relationship. The battle was particularly brutal and the medical staff of the British army was heavily engaged in the days following. After supervising the attentions given to the wounded in the hospitals at Salamanca, McGrigor follows the army's advance to Madrid. On the way, he is appalled by the suffering of the wounded being transported along the line and sends orders to the commissary to provide cars and personnel to assist them. On arriving at headquarters, McGrigor is chastised publicly and violently by Wellington for giving those orders. Wellington thunders, 'I shall be glad to know who is to command the army? I or you? ... As long as you live, sir ... never do anything without my orders.'[17] McGrigor is very shaken by the confrontation. However, the rift between the two is soon made up.

Despite this warning, McGrigor continued to arrange for the evacuation of wounded down the line. In October the army unsuccessfully attempted to besiege Burgos and Wellington was forced to withdraw. As the army began its retreat, Wellington conferred with McGrigor about the position of the sick and wounded, and was pleased to discover that they had already begun to be evacuated via a chain of hospitals from Valladolid to Cuidad Rodrigo and beyond to Oporto. In this 'scene' McGrigor's foresight is praised by Wellington, but McGrigor takes the opportunity to remind him that his initiative on this occasion is no different to that which he had taken at Salamanca.

The retreat was as disorderly and disgraceful to the British army as Moore's retreat to Corunna. However, McGrigor recorded that the medical department were bastions of orderly conduct throughout, and he used the incident to demonstrate the extent to which the medical officers had internalized a military identity, and to which they upheld military values. He reported that Wellington appreciated this and stated that the medical department was 'the only one which [would] obey orders'.[18] He also recorded a 'scene' intended to demonstrate Wellington's regard for him: McGrigor's leg is injured on the retreat, and he is in danger of having to be left behind. On hearing of this Wellington immediately sends his own carriage, the only one in the army, to rescue and transport him.

By the end of the retreat, the privations, exhaustion and exposure suffered by the army had reduced it to a very poor state of health and the medical staff was overwhelmed. Despite McGrigor's requests for more doctors from Britain, the AMB were unable to provide them. To make up the deficiency, McGrigor obtained Wellington's approval to recruit French and Spanish doctors, some from among the prisoners of war. McGrigor is pointed in stating that Wellington supported all his measures to improve the health of the army, and his requests for medical officers from Britain.[19] At this time, Wellington also approved the full execution of McGrigor's 'long-cherished plan of regimental hospitals which [McGrigor] had quietly introduced'[20] and each regiment set about trying to outdo the others by establishing the best and most comfortable hospitals. With this plan now firmly entrenched in the army, McGrigor went on a tour to inspect all the hospitals in January 1813, and issued regulations for the management of regimental hospitals that were specific to the Peninsula service. Wellington also acceded to another of McGrigor's innovations at about this time, the purchase of some portable hospitals for the army, based on the wooden moveable huts McGrigor had seen used for this purpose in the West Indies.

The regimental hospitals were a great success, and large numbers of sick were returned to the army in time for the advance into northern Spain in April 1813. McGrigor records in his diary, 'when we consider that for the last two months no cases have been sent from regiments, the success of the regimental system will be strongly apparent'.[21] During the next campaign in 1814, McGrigor was able to report to the AMB: 'The measure of keeping up the establishment of the regimental hospitals has so greatly tended to render ... army effective that, it has now the fullest sanction of his Excellency the Commander of the Forces'.[22]

At the Battle of Vitoria in June 1814, Wellington gained a key advantage over the French and pushed them back into the Pyrenees. The British pursued them, fighting a series of gruelling battles at a punishing pace and in freezing cold. The army entered France in October and at Toulouse in April 1814, Wellington won the last battle of the Peninsular War. The standard histories record that at Toulouse the army medical service was in the best shape it had ever been and that the surgeons, in particular, were at the height of their practice: 'the wounded had every possible assistance ... and the [medical officers] worked from morning to evening with assiduity. The surgery of the army was at its highest peak of perfection attained during the war.'[23]

The rest of McGrigor's autobiography details his travels in France after the war, the award of his knighthood, and his appointment to the AMB. Throughout, he refers where possible to the continued good relationship he enjoyed with Lord Wellington. Unfortunately, his account does not go into any detail on his years at the AMB nor his work in that role.

McGrigor, Wellington and the New Army Medical Board

It is not the purpose of this chapter to suggest that McGrigor's autobiography is in any way a fiction. However, given his influence on military medicine over the first half of the nineteenth century, a closer analysis of his time in the Peninsula is warranted.

The autobiography, written years after the Wars, makes much of the relationship between McGrigor and Wellington, and historians have frequently commented on their mutual respect and relative closeness. When compared with Wellington's relationship with Dr Franck, it certainly does appear that McGrigor was a 'better fit'. McGrigor's efficient and energetic approach to the administration of his department undoubtedly would have made a favourable impression. Certainly, contemporary sources confirm that McGrigor had constant and sympathetic access to Wellington.[24] Whether the close relationship between the two was unique is less certain. In a study of the administrative arrangements in the Peninsula, Samuel Ward suggests that Wellington pursued a strategy of cultivating close relationships with the heads of all his civil departments. According to Ward, Wellington was very aware of the divided loyalties men such as McGrigor had, as they were answerable to him but also to the heads of their departments at home. His strategy of pursuing close working relationships with all his senior staff was his way of coming between them and their home departments, securing their support, and ensuring he had control over the running of his army.[25] In McGrigor's case, the difficulties he had with the AMB most likely made him a very willing candidate for any such approach by Wellington.

McGrigor's strategy of cultivating the approbation of his commanding military officer to ensure their support for his medical initiatives has already been discussed, and has been noted by other historians. However, in the Peninsula it appears that he also cultivated that relationship in the hope of securing independence from his departmental superiors. Over the course of McGrigor's first year in the Peninsula, his correspondence reveals developing frictions between himself and the AMB. The AMB was obviously keen to keep a very close eye on proceedings in the Peninsula, and attempted to supervise and control McGrigor's command there by questioning his requisitions, querying his plans of treatment and not allowing him to make decisions about promotions within the service. McGrigor's increasing frustration is evident in the tone of his address to the AMB, in his attempts to involve Wellington, and in his asides designed to let the AMB know of the support he was receiving from such a powerful patron.

In April 1812, the AMB wrote McGrigor a letter that closely analysed a return of sickness he had sent them for January and February. The AMB stated that the deaths from fever suffered by the Fusilier Regiment were 'truly lamentable' and asked for the report of the investigation it felt that McGrigor must have undertaken. The AMB also expressed the critical view that 'contagious Typhus is not, or ought not to be, a common disease in an Army (British one at least) in the Field in such a Climate as Portugal'.[26] It also referred to recent reports in a medical publication by a 'highly respectable Medical Officer in the Army in Portugal' claiming the ability to cure dysentery by means of mercury. For this reason, the AMB was 'particularly aggrieved at the number of deaths' from that disease, and stated that it was worse 'than has ever taken place at any preceding period even in climates more unhealthy than Portugal'.[27]

The AMB's criticisms continued over the next few months. They ranged from queries about excessive diets at the general hospitals in Lisbon[28] (reminding him of his duty to observe economy), to dismissing his proposed diet table (stating that wine was known to be bad for health in many circumstances) and strongly suggesting that he use the diet table approved by the AMB in the general and regimental hospitals at home,[29] to subtle suggestions that his medical arrangements were less than optimal. In the AMB's evaluation of his proposed measures to reduce mortality among the troops, it opined that

> The measures recommended by you appear (as far as they go) judicious; and we hope may tend to diminish in some degree the mortality; but the removal of sick labouring under acute diseases from the spot where they are taken ill, to a distant Hospital except even under the most favourable circumstances ... must always tend to aggravate their diseases ... We have therefore to call your attention to our letter of the 10th March on this subject and we feel it our duty to recommend that you represent these circumstances to the Earl of Wellington[30]

This instruction no doubt infuriated McGrigor who had already tried, and failed, to persuade Wellington to allow hospitals to operate nearer the front lines. The AMB did endeavour to meet McGrigor's requests for an augmentation of the medical staff, however it could not resist writing: 'altho' we cannot help entertaining generally the opinion already expressed on several occasions that the provision of Medical Officers for the Service of the Army was adequate to the expected exigencies'.[31]

In the same letter, McGrigor was chastised for recommending certain 'poorly educated' hospital mates for promotion who were 'fit only for the lowest employments in the Hospital'. His ability to evaluate the skill of such men was also called into question, as the AMB felt that they had been 're-examined in Portugal and reports made upon them, which in some instance we have thought were too hastily formed'. It went on to stress that he must make sure the examiners of such men give the matter their greatest care and attention, but that it might be better 'to let all the Hospital Mates abide by the qualifications under which they are sent from England'.[32] McGrigor's tussles with the AMB over promotions were not confined to the matter of the 'defective' hospital mates but, as will be discussed below, extended to his desired promotions of much more senior men. In this context, it is plausible that McGrigor's cultivation of Wellington's patronage was not just a tactic to ensure his plans would be implemented in the Peninsula, but also a recruitment of a powerful ally in his struggle with the AMB for control of what those plans for the medical service would be.

McGrigor used various methods to cultivate the support of Wellington, including highlighting the value of the medical service to the military strength of the army, and closely involving Wellington in his dealings with the AMB. After the siege of Badajoz, McGrigor famously suggested that Wellington commend the medical officers in his dispatch. McGrigor also praised their efforts in his official reports to the AMB, and noted that there had been 'so small a Mortality from among the Wounded'. He further stated that 'a very considerable proportion of the Wounded have been dismissed cured ... and have joined or are on the way to join their Regiments'.[33] This letter was sent to both Wellington and to the AMB, and its emphasis on the returned manpower to Wellington's force demonstrates McGrigor's appreciation of the military utility of his service.

In June 1812, McGrigor drafted a plan to combat the sickness and mortality in the army and submitted it to Wellington. McGrigor used the data he had gathered over the preceding months, and a close analysis of the returns from the 7th and 40th regiments to prove to Wellington that only certain types of soldier should be sent out to the service.[34] In that letter he made several recommendations:

1. Recruits who were underage or incapable of performing the duties of a soldier should not be sent out to the service;
2. the men should be embarked in England in October and if possible gradually inured to marching in the healthier parts of the country;
3. in the colder months in which dysentery and other inflammatory diseases prevailed blankets and great coats should be issued to the men;
4. the balances of payment owed to the men should be gradually paid out instead of being paid in a lump sum;
5. rations should be issued daily; and
6. even though it might have been impossible, McGrigor said it was his duty to suggest again a steady and regular mode of conveying the sick for each brigade.

The plan was reviewed by Wellington and, presumably based on his suggestions, McGrigor submitted an amended version to Lord Liverpool with Wellington's endorsement.[35] Wellington had found the final three suggestions unacceptable, and they were removed. McGrigor's amended letter also contained changes to the other proposals and now suggested sending recruits over in 'December or after the autumnal equinox', and sending troops in clean and airy ships instead of transports. The amended plan was enhanced in other ways; most notably it began by stating McGrigor's claim to expertise, referring to the diseases of the Peninsula as 'so much akin to those of other countries in which I have served'.[36]

Around this time, the AMB escalated its critique of McGrigor's competence, writing to him about his letters on the sickness and mortality prevailing in Coimbra, and suggesting that the buildings must either be in an unhealthy situation, or 'that due attention has not been paid to cleanliness ventilation and diet'. It also expressed the opinion that his report had been very unsatisfactory, that it was 'at a loss to conceive how the Report in its amended state can any more than at first have given satisfaction to Lord Wellington'.[37] McGrigor's response to this affronting suggestion was measured and to the point, but his upset at the AMB's suggestion is plain. However, he clearly re-asserted that Wellington did, in fact, express his approval.[38]

McGrigor also responded to the AMB's criticisms of his requisition of certain necessary articles with a statement that reveals his perception of its opinion of him:

> It is a matter of regret to me that the Board should think I inconsiderately call for stores which cannot be converted to use in any instance ... It has been my wish to act so as to obtain the Confidence and support of the Board.[39]

In a letter on the same matter he defended himself from accusations that he had unnecessarily involved Wellington, 'It was not from my suggestion, but from his own observation, that Lord Wellington wrote to the Secretary at War'. He went on to make his position clear:

> It is painful to me, that in the execution of my duty, I should have merited your disapprobation or displeasure, because, from the moment of my arrival in this Country, I have been studiously anxious to act in strict conformity to your orders ... and I had even flattered myself, that I was entitled to the same approbation from you, which His Excellency the Commander of the Forces here has on more than one occasion been pleased to bestow on my arrangements and exertions. I would even hope, that with the local knowledge, as His Lordship possesses you would not disapprove of any proceeding of mine ...
>
> I can only add that if you will be pleased to point out to me any line of conduct I will endeavour to follow it, in the execution of duty and if you grant me the same confidence and support which His Excellency the Commander of the Forces and his family [continues] to me here the service will continue to be conducted to the credit of the Department and to the advantage of the public.[40]

In that letter McGrigor firmly positioned himself behind the support of Lord Wellington, and implied that the Board were behaving unreasonably and in contradiction of Wellington's aims, wisdom, and local knowledge. The Board's response shows it perceived the potential damage from such implications, and that it also was not above drawing senior military figures into the matter:

> [we] must express some little surprize [*sic*] at the tone of your Letter; as we are certainly not aware of having expressed any thing like disapprobation or displeasure or shewn a want of confidence in your zeal, talents and exertions or of withholding any support which it could be in our power to afford you; towards the due execution of the arduous and important service in which you are engaged.
>
> Thinking your remonstrance very serious we have thought it incumbent on us to give a statement of the circumstances to the secretary at War to remove from his Lordship's mind, as well as from the Marquis of Wellington, any impression they might have received of our having a wish to restrict you in the proper supplies for the service of the army[41]

McGrigor also used non-confrontational letters to let the AMB know of his strong position in the Peninsula. He had always been assiduous in commending medical officers for their good works, and in ensuring that his good reports of them were received not only by the AMB but also by military commanders. In his letters to the AMB from this time commending various officers for their good works he began to make subtle aversions about Wellington's satisfaction with himself and his department. In July 1812, McGrigor wrote:

> His Excellency the Commander of the Forces has been pleased to direct that the very favourable reports made to him by the General Officers who visited the stations at Badajoz, Abrantes, Santarem, Celerico, Castello Branco and Viza should be shewn to me[42]

At the same time, McGrigor was writing to Wellington, emphasizing his own hard work, and referring to the obstructions the AMB was putting in the way of them achieving their goals. He solicited Wellington's assistance in forcing the AMB to do what he wanted:

> I have endeavoured to make the best arrangement for the Wounded ... From the great fatigue of duty, as well as from Illness the Medical Officers are much wanted for which I made requisition on the Medical Board some time ago and I beg here to suggest to your Lordship that the Board be called up by the Commander in Chief to order them out immediately.[43]

McGrigor also sought to assert his dominance over the AMB on the issue of promotions. His efforts to have certain officers promoted caused problems with the AMB, and again McGrigor drew Wellington into the dispute. One of the officers that McGrigor and Wellington sought to promote was Mr John Gunning, nephew of the former surgeon general of the same name.[44] Wellington and McGrigor petitioned repeatedly for Gunning's promotion but Weir was unable to persuade the Duke of York to accede to their request.[45]

It appears that McGrigor and Wellington decided to promote Gunning in any event, and on 27 September, McGrigor wrote to say that 'His Excellency the Commander of the Forces has been pleased to Appoint Staff Surgeon John Gunning to be acting Surgeon Major to the Forces in the Peninsula ... from the 22nd Inst'.[46]

Soon after (and probably before that letter was received) Gunning was appointed a deputy inspector of hospitals.[47] Other disputes over promotion were not resolved as easily. Weir continued to assert his right to control promotions within the army, often turning down those McGrigor recommended. When McGrigor raised objections about this he was accused of 'presuming to question [Weir's] objections', which of course he denied. Instead McGrigor repeatedly pointed to the good reports made by senior medical officers in the Peninsula about those he had sought to promote, and never failed to mention Wellington's interest in the matter:

> several medical officers have now testified to the great improvement Mr Starr has made particularly Staff Surgeon Hennen. From Mr Starr's extraordinary zeal and attention, which I frequently witnessed and which his Excellency the Commander of the Forces noticed at Elvas I was induced specially to recommend him at the time.[48]

McGrigor also requested permission to examine hospital mates for promotion in the Peninsula, instead of sending them back to England for the purpose.[49] He referred to his own observations of the men he tried to advance, and detailed their claims to promotion based on what they had done in the Peninsula. He asked Weir:

> As then these Officers have reason to believe that they are qualified for promotion, and as they know that strong statements of their merits have been transmitted to me by the inspection officers under whom they have served I request you will be pleased to inform me what answer I am to make to the many letters which they write me on the subject of their promotion[50]

Throughout his first year in the Peninsula, McGrigor had been repeatedly petitioning the Board for more medical staff, and for the return of the medical staff he believed were lingering on leave in England without due cause. Wellington had been very supportive of McGrigor in this matter, but the Board insisted that it did not believe more men were necessary, McGrigor's calculations about the men remaining in England were wrong, and that even if it had wanted to send him more medical officers, there were none to send. McGrigor persisted in his requests and wrote official letters to Wellington and to other senior military officers. McGrigor's representations in this regard became offensive to the Board and they cautioned him:

We are persuaded that in the hurry of writing you have not attended so much as might be wished to the import of a word, or weighed the effects that such assertions may have on the minds of those to whom they are made. In every estimate allowances must be made for sickness, and the officers who are absent from Duty, on that account, can never, with any degree of propriety, be reckoned among the deficiencies. When replying to the adjutant general we felt it necessary to bring this point particularly under notice; and we have presented to the Commander in Chief, through the military secretary, as well as through the adjutant general, abstracts to shew the actual state of the general and regimental medical staff under your orders ...

In replying to the Commander in Chief we were impelled to express our surprise at the manner in which you had addressed the Marquis of Wellington earnestly and anxiously hoping that 'Promotion may go to those only who have been actually serving on the spot' whenever a fresh staff is found for foreign service or an augmentation made to one already employed it is imperative on us to employ those officer who are at home on the half pay or unattached before the country can be burthened [*sic*] by new appointments; but assuredly the instances of four Deputy Inspectors, two Physicians, ten or twelve Staff Surgeons, three apothecaries and eight deputy purveyors; besides all vacancies of Regimental and Assistant Surgeons that happen, may be taken in proof that little or no obstruction has been made to the Recommendations sent home through the commander of the forces[51]

This very explicit letter did not cause McGrigor to back down. Instead, he took the AMB on over his desired promotion of Dr Charles Tice and Surgeon George Guthrie both to the rank of deputy inspector of hospitals. Weir refused to promote either of them because 'dissatisfaction would be created by the promotion of two officers of ... short services', and also because the Duke of York had directed that a different deputy inspector should be appointed and staff surgeon promoted. Weir tried to make the best of it by noting that the staff surgeon in question had previously been recommended by Wellington.[52] In response, McGrigor wrote Wellington the most extraordinary letter (set out here in full because of its importance):

It is painful to me to be obliged to intrude on your Lordship's time and attention at a moment when I know they are engaged with the most important concerns. Nothing but my conviction that the Department, which I have the honor to superintend in your Lordship's Army is about to suffer a most serious injury, unless your Lordship [interfere] could have induced me to intrude at this time.

By an official communication which I have just received from the Army Medical Board, I learn, that the Director General not only refuses to confirm your Lordships recommendation of Dr. Tice and Mr Guthrie to be Deputy Inspectors of Hospitals, but has determined to fill up the vacancies occasioned by the deaths of Dr. Gray and Mr — by the appointment of Mr Higgins and Mr Taylor a Deputy Inspector from the home service.

As we lost these valuable officers in the active and zealous performance of their duties here; I did hope that no attempt would be made to fill up these vacancies, occasioned by their deaths, but from any officers equally distinguished for zeal and ability, in the same army.

I do earnestly intreat [*sic*] your Lordship's protection for the staff, and interposition to prevent a most serious injury, not to Messers Tice and Guthrie alone, but to the body of officers on the service, who animated by your Lordship's approbation have displayed an extraordinary degree of zeal.

Dr. Tice has with diligence and admirable system regulated the Hospitals at Celerico, Coimbra and the intermediate stations: he has introduced order where none existed before, and brought stations whence produced the greatest mortality to be among the most healthy.

Mr Guthrie is one of the ablest Surgeons and best medical officers in the service: his exertions during the siege of Badajos and after the battle of 22nd July, and his arrangements at Salamanca did him the greatest credit and really are beyond praise.

The merits of Deputy Inspector Taylor are unknown to me, and whatever Mr Higgins' claims may have been, he appears to me to have forfeited them by deserting this Army in quest of promotion for upwards of a year, and remaining at home at the most critical period.

I do not wish to derogate from the merits of any man. I only wish to vindicate the rights of the Medical Staff of this Army: if these two Gentlemen have claims for promotion and employment I hope the Director General will find employment for them on other services, without — on the rights of those who have been unceasingly employed under your Lordship.

It really has been my most anxious wish and highest ambition to obtain your Lordship's confidence, and your approbation of the Medical Department. Flattered as I have been by your notice of them, and seeing the Officers of the Department most animated to fresh exertions by this notice, I would deeply deplore the occurrence of anything that could damp their zeal, or slacken their exertions, and I much fear that this threatened act and intrusion would have this evil tendency.

I feel an affection for the service and my own Department noticed as it has been by your Lordship. I am therefore induced earnestly to entreat that you will kindly interfere for those who look up to your Lordship as their protector.[53]

This is not only of interest because of its blatant appeal for Wellington's assistance and its characterization of the AMB as an entity operating against the interests of the British army, but also for the matters that McGrigor chose to highlight to Wellington in describing the medical staff. He begins the letter by emphasizing their military honours, noting that the two officers to be replaced had died in the performance of their duties, and implies that their successors should be men who had bravely exposed themselves to the same risks. The professional qualifications of both Tice and Guthrie are stressed, but moreover Tice's success in bringing 'order' to the hospitals and returning fighting strength to the army is highlighted, as is Guthrie's battle experience at the siege of Badajoz. Hence McGrigor emphasized the military benefits these officers had provided, as well as their own militaristic qualities. The loyalty of the medical staff as a whole is drawn out, and contrasted with the cowardly and disloyal actions of Dr Higgins who remained at home during a 'most critical period'. Above all, McGrigor's letter sets his medical staff apart from the AMD at home, and emphasizes its quality as a unit integrated by bonds of loyalty and valour into Wellington's army. In these ways, his appeal not only requests Wellington's help, but makes a clear statement about the militarization of his staff whose first loyalty is to the army, which the army should reciprocate.

Through the use of all these methods, McGrigor had successfully enlisted Wellington as an ally in his struggle against the superintendence of the AMB. Blanco demonstrates that Wellington had been making representations against the AMB's promotion policy to Lord Bathurst and to Colonel Henry Torrens.[54] Unfortunately, the AMB's response to this campaign is not contained in any official record and the outcome of this dispute over promotions policy is not clear. It appears, however, that McGrigor won the day, as Tice and Guthrie were promoted in 1813[55] and after this time the AMB adopted a less critical and interventionist approach to McGrigor's administration.

McGrigor and His Staff

McGrigor's perception of the medical staff in the Peninsula as a distinct and separate body was not one he only adopted as a strategy to impress Wellington. In his letters about and to his staff he adopted the tone of a firm parent, and sought to strengthen the bond between himself and his men by always praising their good work and letting them know he had drawn it to the attention of senior military officers.[56] In his letters he not only praised the achievements of his staff, but linked those achievements to the performance of the army: 'The service owes very much to Deputy Inspector Robb and to Acting Deputy Inspector Tice for the excellent state into which the Hospitals have been brought'.[57]

He also emphasized another key aspect of the military medical officer identity – their dual expertise as both surgeons and physicians:

> Since the illness of Staff Surgeon — Dr. Neale [a physician] has not only done all the ordinary Surgical Duties; but has performed amputation and other surgical operations whenever they were required.[58]

After the Battle of Toulouse, McGrigor sent an official letter of farewell to his staff, through the principal medical officers at the stations in Portugal and Spain. In the letter he drew together all these themes referring to the 'tie' that had developed between himself and his medical staff. He referred to the trying circumstances in which they had all struggled, and in which they had overcome much together. In particular, he expressed his gratitude for the support that those gentlemen had given him and without which he said he could 'never have conducted the duties with either satisfaction to myself or advantage to the

public'. He also asked the senior medical officers to communicate his approbation of the junior officers to them, and was particular to name those who had
come to his personal attention. At the end of the letter, he reported that he had
communicated his assessments of those officers to both the AMB and the commander of the forces. In this way, McGrigor continued the art, which he had
perfected during the Peninsular War, of forming links between disparate groups,
and between the military and medical departments of the army. This letter gives
the impression that McGrigor genuinely cared about the 'family' of medical
officers he had created, but also that he was intent on promoting in those men
a particular vocabulary and way of thinking about their service. The letter was
intended to reach the ears, if not the eyes, of every medical officer in the army
and the terms in which it was written characterized those men not just as medical professionals, but as military officers who had contributed to the success of
the army and as public servants who had performed great acts of valour for their
country.[59] McGrigor had spent much of his time advancing that multi-layered
character of military medical officers to those outside the medical service, and
now he was arming his medical officers with the same language with which to
represent themselves.

Medicine in the Peninsula

McGrigor's perception of the service as a particularly 'military medicine', was
also reflected in the practice of medicine that he encouraged in the Peninsula.
His most noted reform (and probably the most efficacious) was the rigid enforcement of a hygienic order: inspection of soldiers; airy hospital wards; and the
separation of diseases into different classes and wards. These were measures that
lent themselves to military enforcement, and because of their orderly structure
probably also appealed to military minds.[60] In addition to this natural appeal,
McGrigor took every opportunity to remind Wellington of the importance of
such measures, drilling home his views on the causes and nature of disease.[61]
His relentless pursuit of a system of regimental hospitals, which so effectively
stopped the constant movement of slight cases to the rear, was 'military' not
just in its aim of returning fighting men to the front as soon as possible, but also
in the values he articulated in the support of the plan. The emphasis that advocates of the regimental system placed on the notion that military discipline and
camaraderie within a regiment was essential to the restoration of health demonstrated their 'understanding' of the ways of the soldier and also articulated their
support of such regimental bonds. These aspects of McGrigor's administration
in the Peninsula have been extensively reported by medical historians. However,
McGrigor's clinical endeavours have received less attention. The military appeal
of his hygienic measures is obvious, and was no doubt very useful in recruiting

Wellington to his cause. The clinical approach he took in his administration was also likely to have had a similar effect.

Despite the multiplicity of treatments commonly used for various diseases, McGrigor believed that there was such a thing as 'best practice'. He worked hard to divine what this was and to disseminate this knowledge amongst his staff. In that process, the observations of disease and treatment he requested to accompany statistical returns from medical officers were just as important as the numbers of sick and killed they gave him. McGrigor's continued reliance on the collection, collation and distribution of information from his medical officers, developed in Egypt, continued to inform his medical administration in the Peninsula. His 'private journal' includes copious notes taken from the reports he had received on the various treatments that were being used, particularly for dysentery and fever, throughout the Peninsula.[62] He gave extensive detail about the work of individual practitioners in his paper on the medical history of the British army in the Peninsula, written just after the conclusion of the Wars.[63] In addition to creating a sense of imagined community amongst the practitioners in the Peninsula, this process also enabled McGrigor to advocate certain practices over others. His methods of doing so were quite subtle, often taking the form only of his reporting on the success of a particular officer, but it does appear that they were effective and in some diseases he was able to report to the AMB a consensus about treatment across his staff. For example: 'the well known and established practice of using Mercury in Dysentery as lately recommended by Mr Fergusson is in use in the Hospitals on this service'.[64]

His post-war report given to the medico-chirurgical society also demonstrates a higher level of consistent practice in the Peninsula than on other campaigns. In his discussion of the 'infinite' varieties of fever faced by the medical staff, there is not a great deal of variety in the treatments which he reports were attempted.[65] From his report it appears that some success was achieved with stimulants, sudorifics, Peruvian bark, the warm bath and blisters, but that treatment with cold affusions and purgatives was likely to do harm. In mild cases his report implies that the shaving of heads, application of leeches and the use of blisters was widespread and successful. His report is similarly indicative of a widespread practice in the treatment of remittent fever with cold affusions and bleeding, and in intermittent fever with the use of bark, bleeding and cold affusions. In the case of dysentery he reports a definite consensus of practice: 'to attack the disease vigorously by depletion on its earliest commencement'.[66] He had seen the good effects of this practice in Portsmouth in 1810 and 1811, and 'the plan of Dr. Somers appeared so judicious ... that I recommended its being generally followed in the army'.[67] Similarly, he reports that in cases of pneumonia the only appropriate remedy was the lancet.[68]

That he attempted to bring about this type of consensus among his staff can be ascertained from several strategies he adopted. The most overt was his attempt to both improve and standardize the practice of medicine in the Peninsula through the ongoing education of young medical officers by senior mentors that he appointed. In this regard he was particularly anxious to have Dr Somers appointed as physician in chief to the army:

> the professional ability of Dr. Somers, and his long experience ... might be very usefully applied to the benefit of the service, — sending him to the principal Hospital Stations where there is much disease or considerable mortality, at several of the stations he could with much advantage regulate the practice of the junior Medical Officers with this service.[69]

He explained to the AMB a few weeks later that Wellington had made the appointment until the pleasure of the Prince Regent was known and that

> Dr. Somers, who is senior Physician in the Army, of late [has] been exerting himself very zealously, and it is my intention to employ him occasionally at different Hospital Stations in correcting the practice of the Junior Medical Officers, in same manner as Mr Gunning will act regarding the surgical practices.[70]

The same intention is evident in his regulations issued for the regulation of general hospitals on the service, which include an exhortation on senior medical officers to train junior officers and also a requirement to report to McGrigor about the progress of those students.[71] This requirement was repeated in the rules concerning reports and followed by the caution that:

> 60. It is to be generally understood, that the Inspector of Hospitals is principally guided in his recommendations for promotion, by these reports, and by no means, by mere seniority.[72]

Within regimental hospitals, confidential reports on the educational attainments and progress of junior medical officers were also demanded, and the obligation to train younger medical officers was thought to be even more serious.[73] The regulations included a formulary which specified the treatments that were to be used in the hospitals, but also incorporated McGrigor's consultative approach to the discovery of the best treatments:

> 109. A formulary of medicine for the use of all hospitals on this service having been prepared and arranged from the communications and experience of the medical officers, it is to be observed throughout all hospitals general and regimental. It being intended annually to correct this formulary, in order to include all improvements, which experience may prove to be advantageous. Communications from the senior officers and particularly from the Physicians of the army, are requested on this subject.[74]

The likelihood of a junior medical officer deciding to deviate from what McGrigor considered 'best practice' in these circumstances, seems remote. When different treatments were tried, McGrigor was vigilant in supervising the outcome:

> It is very desirable that an eye be kept on the cases of Hospital Gangrene which has been treated at — by SS Burmeister, and that the final result of each be known. This mode of treatment is at variance with that which has ultimately been found successful in most of the Hospitals in the Peninsula.[75]

The overwhelming majority of treatments advocated by McGrigor were cost efficient. Bleeding, cold water dousing and blistering were his most commonly recommended treatments and, as has already been noted, these were particularly suited to military notions of manliness. But not all diseases yielded readily to these methods, and as in Egypt, McGrigor encouraged the systematic use of trial and experiment to find cures for those that did not. It has been noted that military authorities were most interested in specific cures capable of application to large populations of sick,[76] and the trials conducted by McGrigor in the Peninsula support this observation. Some trials on the Peninsular sick were directed by the AMB. In particular, the AMB instructed McGrigor to make trials of a 'bark gingerbread' that had been extensively considered in Britain, which made use of damaged bark. In 1812, the AMB wrote to McGrigor about the gingerbread, stating that Doctor Robertson, at the Royal Hospital at Greenwich had urged them to trial it, and now they forwarded some to him to 'trial on the army of the Peninsula'.[77] McGrigor also instituted a trial of different types of bark in intermittent fever,[78] and oversaw the wide variety of unsuccessful therapies that were attempted in the cure of tetanus.[79] In the latter case McGrigor regretted 'that the method of cure is yet to be discovered' but noted that the hundreds of cases and extensive trials had made an important contribution to medicine generally: 'In pointing out what military practice has enabled us to do, towards ascertaining the effects of medicines in large doses, and carried to their ultimate extent, I hope to leave the ground more open for the trial of new remedies'.[80]

In the foregoing analysis of McGrigor's approach to the treatment of disease in the Peninsula his 'militarization' of the medical staff is clear. The treatments he was most supportive of were likely to appeal to military officers because of their low cost and logistic adaptability, as well as for aesthetic reasons. Moreover, his emphasis on the provision of treatment in regimental hospitals ensured that military commanders were made familiar with the methods of treatment adopted. His emphasis on training junior officers, keeping their practice under close surveillance, and providing reports on their progress all replicated military command structures and further integrated medical officers into a military institution, distinct from autonomous civilian practice.

In total, his hygienic reforms, rhetoric and practice in the pursuit of regimental hospitals, militaristic therapies, training and reporting systems, praise of the bravery and valour of his staff, and his continued operation as a 'hub and disseminator' of medical information, all contributed to the creation of a medical service that perceived itself to be a distinct community which was thoroughly integrated into, and contributing to, the success of Wellington's army.

Officers and Gentlemen

The effects of all McGrigor's efforts in this direction were profound but they were not the sole force pushing the medical staff towards a militarized professional identity. Much of the impetus for military integration appears to have come from the medical officers themselves. The appeal of military service to young medical officers such as Dent has already been noted, and it seems that the attractions it held did not erode with time. Towards the end of the Wars, Dent wrote to his cousin rejecting the idea of settling down to private practice, which he believed would primarily involve 'running fidgeting after a parcel of old Women'.[81] A similar picture was painted by one of his contemporaries, who foresaw the competition that would prevail within profession after the peace:

> Napoleon's return was a good thing for me; inasmuch as, the next economical proceeding to be performed by the Government was a further reduction of the Army, and I should have been relegated to half pay, and earning guineas by insinuating myself into the good graces of desponding old maids with chronic coughs and asthmas, and of crusty old bachelors, victims to living not wisely but too well.[82]

The similar language used in these separate accounts suggests that such characterizations of civilian practice were common parlance among the medical officers serving under McGrigor. Such characterizations emphasized the feminized, geriatric and obsequious aspects of private practice and in their disparagement of them implied a strong preference for military culture and military patients.[83] The advantages of treating military patients may have been related to the nature of their diseases, their forced compliance, or any other number of factors; the preference for a military lifestyle probably related to the particular nature of the bonds that were formed by these men while on service.

It certainly appears that the attachments that were formed among regimental brothers were extended to and very much valued by medical officers. Regimental medical officers shared the privations and travails of their regiments and, perhaps unsurprisingly, often described themselves as one of the men. The bonds that were created by such shared experiences are evocatively described by Gibney:

> For many years they had lived together, shared privations, hardships, and dangers; the regiment was the only home they knew, and now this was broken up. In more respects

than one the partings resembled the wrench to family ties caused by marriage, death, or certain incidents occurring in everyday life.[84]

The bonds between regimental brothers were also probably exhibited most poignantly in the regimental hospitals:

> Those comforts, which at home are sure to be provided for the chamber of an invalid are wanting. Yet, here, some warm-hearted friend will smooth the pillow for your feverish head, will speak to you in the manly yet feeling language of encouragement; will procure, and often prepare for you some delicacy; and, in the dark and silent hour of evening will sit quietly by your side, consoling you by affectionate pressures of the hand, for pain and suffering, and watching anxiously that nothing may interrupt or scare your needful slumbers, Yes, – such a picture is not romantic; in civil life, men have homes, parents, wives, children, brothers, sister; but in the profession of arms they become dependant on friends. No where is friendship more true, more warm, more exalted, than in the army; absence from the mother-country, privation, peril, the pursuit and attainment of honor, are so many ties which bind soul to soul, in bonds bright and Indestructible.[85]

Both during and after the Wars, many medical officers published observations or diaries of their time in the Peninsula. Rosner has noted that these works, and also the letters of Peninsula medical officers, are remarkably deficient in descriptions of medical practice.[86] Overwhelmingly, they instead present a portrait of themselves as participants in the army as officers and gentlemen. The conclusion to be drawn from these works is not that medical officers did not care about their medical work, but that the public face they wished to present was a military one. In this regard we can refer especially to the books written by Halliday and Neale which touched almost not at all on medicine, and instead were very much directed at the reporting and analysis of military operations.[87] Even in his work on the Portuguese army, Halliday only devoted a small proportion of his analysis to the medical department.[88] Similarly, the works of Boutflower,[89] Thomson,[90] Broughton,[91] Henry,[92] and James[93] focus on the day-to-day events of military life, the quality of billets, some heroics, the local women and the description of battles in which they were engaged. In writing these memoirs the aspirations of medical officers to a gentlemanly status is also evident in their frequent adoption of the picturesque to describe the vistas of Portugal or the sites of battles.[94]

By the end of the Peninsular War, it is evident that the medical staff viewed themselves as military officers, and that they were practising a distinctly militarized medicine. They had embraced the culture and values of regimental life, were largely reconciled to command structures and subordination even as it related to their medical practice, aspired to gentlemanly status as officers not just as practitioners, had adopted a vocabulary in which their services were represented as contributing to the success of the army, and were desirous of being acknowledged for both their medical and military achievements. The published recollections of many medical officers promoted all these aspects of their service, as did McGrigor in the first years of his appointment to the AMB.

Conclusion

This chapter has endeavoured to provide a more critical portrait of McGrigor and his work in the Peninsular War than has previously been attempted. It is clear that he made significant efforts to develop a close working relationship with Wellington, both to smooth the implementation of his administrative and medical reforms, and to help dilute the control of the AMB over him. McGrigor employed a variety of tactics to achieve this goal: providing a medicine that was efficient and logistically adaptable; educating and consulting Wellington about medical matters; representing the AMB as their common adversary; enforcing military command structures within the medical department; advertising the military utility of the medical service; and extolling the militaristic virtues of the medical staff. McGrigor also cultivated the approbation of military officers further down the chain of command, demonstrating his sophisticated understanding of the environment in which he was working. Many of these tactics had the additional effect of further promoting a culture that had developed amongst the medical staff in which they saw themselves as both military officers and medical practitioners. His administration also oversaw the achievement of a greater consensus amongst the medical staff on therapeutics than had been achieved previously in the Wars, which contributed further to the medical staff's belief that they were distinct from and more expert than their civilian counterparts. As has been demonstrated in previous chapters, the distinctness and expertise of military medical practitioners had been a topic of fierce debate from the beginning of the Wars. After the Peninsular War the issue was to be raised again, and even debated in Parliament. McGrigor's central role in this debate is considered in the following chapter.

6 BEYOND THE WARS

The professional identity and medical practice of the medical officers of the British army had changed significantly between the outbreak of war in 1793 and the Battle of Waterloo in 1815. This chapter will demonstrate that the military medicine they practised was a significant force in the development of British medicine more generally in the years following the Wars.

It is now clear that the emergence of hospital medicine in France owed much to military medicine. However, the transition to hospital medicine in Britain is generally acknowledged to have developed more gradually than on the Continent and to have been influenced by a wide variety of changes within a vibrant 'medical marketplace' where older models continued to exist alongside hospital medicine for a much longer period. The militarized medicine that had been embraced by British military medical officers shared many characteristics with hospital medicine, particularly the exertion of control over patients, the classification and segregation of different disease and surgical classes, and an ontological, lesion-based understanding of disease. As they flooded back into the civilian marketplace, British medical officers helped to bring this type of medicine to their patients and communities. At the same time, British medicine experienced the rise of the general practitioner, a professional identity that blurred the traditional line between physic and surgery that the military medical officer also advocated.

The benefits of military medicine to the general community were also advocated from within the AMD where McGrigor presided over the promotion of the discoveries and achievements of his medical officers. Finally, military medical officers pursued claims of expertise in heated debates thrashed out in parliamentary select committees of inquiry. Through this dual process of assimilation and advocacy, British military medical officers made a significant contribution to the development of medicine in Britain in the first half of the nineteenth century. They were important agents in the production of a culture that was receptive to hospital medicine.

Demobilization and Civilian Practice

After the Wars, the AMD was rapidly demobilized and a flood of military practitioners descended upon the British civilian marketplace. Ackroyd et al., estimate that over the years 1816–23 approximately 700 army surgeons would have attempted to enter civilian practice in Britain. Together with their naval colleagues these men represented an increase of 5–6 per cent to the civilian profession.[1] In the same study the authors also demonstrate that although many encountered difficulties in setting up practice, a significant proportion went on to establish successful civilian careers. They conclude 'It is clear, too, that many made a great success of their civilian practice ... there is sufficient evidence to suggest many not only prospered but also continued to contribute to practice and medical knowledge particularly as teachers and hospital doctors'.[2] Given the length of service many of these practitioners had given to the army, and the widespread adoption by army practitioners of the particular medical philosophy detailed in previous chapters, it is reasonable to assume that these practitioners carried aspects of military medicine with them into civilian practice, and into any teaching they undertook. In 1819, the physician Benjamin Welsh observed in a study on venesection, that demobilized army and navy practitioners had 'settled in almost every corner of the empire ... generally carrying along with them the practice which they have hitherto found so beneficial'.[3]

Many found a ready base for their practice in the spa towns such as Cheltenham where centres for the treatment of tropical invalids had been established. These returned invalids and retirees from the colonies were likely to have been predisposed to the style of medicine practised by ex-army and East India Company doctors, and certainly many practitioners who set up business in these areas thrived.[4] These practitioners applied the expertise they had developed in tropical countries, and the prevailing treatment for the largely bilious complaints of the invalids who frequented these centres was based on a purgative regime revolving around calomel and the mineral waters of the spas. These towns were frequented by thousands of visitors and patients each year, which meant that the ex-military practitioners practising there had a significant audience for the display of their skills and expertise. While the effect of this exposure would have gone some way to promote military medicine within the wider community, it must be remembered that as the majority of the invalids formed part of an ex-military community themselves, the effect of these centres on the dissemination and promotion of the expertise of military practitioners among the general population was probably limited.

Greater effect was achieved by the widespread adoption of therapeutics advocated by the AMD. As seen in the spa towns, ex-military practitioners considered that the approach to the treatment of disease they had learned on service was suitable for civilians, although many felt it was necessary to temper the severity of certain treatments to allow for the less robust constitution of their new patients. A clear example of the influence of military therapeutics is provided by the proliferation of the use of venesection in the twenty years following the Wars. As described in Chapter 3, the innovation of treating Egyptian ophthalmia with aggressive bloodletting had been adopted for the treatment of civilian patients suffering the same disease, albeit in a more moderate form. Copious bloodletting continued to be favoured in military practice throughout the first quarter of the nineteenth century, particularly in the treatment of inflammatory diseases, fever and pneumonia. As Neibyl has demonstrated, ex-military practitioners engaged in civilian practice in Britain and elsewhere around the globe persisted with the therapy and brought about what he termed a 'bloodletting revolution' whereby the treatment came back into vogue for a time.[5]

According to Welsh, military practitioners had promoted this approach through official communications, letters written to medical journals and in MD dissertations.[6] Niebyl's research also makes clear that many of the practitioners who were advocating venesection were working in, or heading, fever hospitals in Britain. There they were able to observe large populations of patients and use the statistics they could derive from those observations to help prove their case. In so doing, they not only helped to promote their therapies, but also the tools of analysis and evidence that were central to the military and 'hospital' approaches to medicine. The influence that could be derived from a hospital post lay both in the ability to treat, and report on the treatment of, large numbers of patients suffering broadly the same diseases, but also in the opportunity it provided to impart knowledge to the medical students who attended the hospitals as part of their training. Military practitioners who returned to civilian practice considered themselves well qualified to head fever hospitals, dispensaries and asylums and they were quite successful in obtaining these posts. Roughly 20 per cent who returned to the United Kingdom secured hospital appointments, which was no insignificant achievement and testifies to the esteem in which their skills were held by the medical societies in which they practised.[7] In order to obtain such posts, practitioners were required to give an account of their skills and learning, and through that forum they were able to argue for the importance and relevance of their military experience. William Fergusson argued strongly that his military experience gave him a greater understanding of fevers and their treatment than he could ever have gained in civilian practice, thereby hoping to bolster his application for one such post.[8] In these positions they would have had control over the treatment of large numbers of patients, and also the responsibility for teaching newcomers to the profession. The example of bloodletting shows that military practitioners were able to use the tools at their disposal to disseminate aspects of their approach throughout the British medical community, and that that community was receptive to it. Given the breadth of topics on which they also wrote to the medical journals it is fair to assume that other aspects of military medicine, including the arrangement of hospitals, understanding of disease and less tangible notions such as a more authoritative dynamic between doctor and patient were also passed on.

In all these ways we can see that in the dispersion of ex-military practitioners throughout the British medical community the military medicine they had developed and practised during the Wars was not abandoned in their treatment of civilian patients, and that they had ample opportunity to promote their approach both within the profession and to their students. It is also unlikely that they were able to completely shed the authoritative approach to the doctor/patient dynamic they had enjoyed during the Wars, and that was also characteristic of the newly emergent hospital medicine. The subtle effect of this dispersion within the civilian market strongly supported the values and patient expectations that underpinned the emergence of hospital medicine in Britain, and to some extent, also the concurrent rise of the general practitioner.

The Army Medical Department

The case for the returned army medical practitioners was also trumpeted from within the AMD. McGrigor, now director general, was tireless in his efforts to promote the service, expertise and social status of both those who remained in his department and decommissioned medical officers who tried to make their way in the civilian marketplace.

Some of McGrigor's efforts to improve the reputation and practice of military medicine after the Wars are well known. In particular, he is credited with continuing to improve the medical care given to the rank and file by encouraging army medical officers to pursue further study and holding out the assurance that further promotion would be based on educational accomplishments and demonstrated abilities. To this end, he was also instrumental in establishing two chairs of military surgery at the universities of Edinburgh and Dublin. Most significantly, his passion for the value of accumulated knowledge and the power of statistics to reveal medical facts was realized when in 1837 Henry Marshall (an ex-military medical officer) and Lt Alexander Murray Tulloch produced *The Statistical Report on the Sickness, Mortality, and Invaliding Among the Troops in the West Indies* based on some of the 160 volumes of returns that McGrigor had solicited from medical officers stationed all over the globe for just such a purpose.[9]

These achievements have been acclaimed by historians for the benefits they were intended to bestow on the rank and file of the army, and for the successes McGrigor had in this despite the failure of the AMD to respond adequately to the challenges of the Crimean War just four years after McGrigor's retirement.

The effect of McGrigor's efforts on the promotion of military medicine outside the service and his advocacy of the benefits it could give to civilian medicine has not received the same attention. The contribution of the *Statistical Report* has certainly not gone unnoticed as an important step in the rise of statistical analysis as a medical tool, and at the time it was credited by mainstream journals such as the *Quarterly Review* for bestowing 'the most valuable gifts, as to the effect of climate, which has ever been made to medicine'.[10] However, right from the start of his tenure at the head of the AMD, McGrigor was also working hard to promote the achievements and skills of his men to Parliament and to the public in general.

He was cognizant of the benefit that would accrue to the service if the heroic efforts of his officers were made known to the public. In this regard he encouraged the publication of several tracts about the Battle of Waterloo by military medical officers. He wrote to one correspondent: 'I am ready at all times to give any aid to you, or any Gentleman ... in giving to the medical world, the medical history of the memorable victory of Waterloo',[11] and believed that it would be best if the works were published before 'the warm feelings exacted by [recollections of the battle] in the public mind have cooled'.[12]

As shown in previous chapters, McGrigor himself published several accounts of the achievements of the AMD after the Wars. These works were intended for a wide audience and demonstrate McGrigor's desire to promote the medical officers of the army as able practitioners with an expertise extending beyond the confines of traditional divisions between surgery and medicine, to whom the public were indebted, and who moreover had a special understanding of disease. His 'Sketch of the Medical History of the British Armies in the Peninsula of Spain and Portugal' was presented to a distinguished medical audience shortly after the peace. He used the paper to not only establish the success of his work in the Peninsula, but also more generally to set forth claims that great improvements had been made in military medicine in the preceding twenty years.[13] In doing so he emphasized the nature of military practice, and pointed out that many discoveries had been made by practitioners in the navy and army, 'by experience and observation'.[14] In this way, McGrigor went about promoting the educational model by which many army medical practitioners had gained their expertise. This was to become very important in the debates which were later aired in Parliament, and which are discussed later in this chapter.

In addition to the well-known efforts McGrigor made to encourage medical officers to pursue opportunities for further medical education following the peace, he also set about disseminating the accumulated medical experience and findings the medical department had gathered during the Wars. In his new position, McGrigor was able to amplify the same techniques he had used on the service to facilitate the transfer of medical information. Once again taking on the role of a 'hub', McGrigor was eager to forward the enquiries of prominent medical men about certain diseases to the medical men who remained in the Peninsula and on station elsewhere around the globe.[15] He also made the public documents of the medical department open to any 'professional gentleman' who might wish to consult them.[16]

One of the most important medical innovations to come out of the Peninsular War was the Portuguese treatment of syphilis without mercury. Fergusson had written about the treatment soon after observing it, and while quite supportive of it he expressed some reservation about the likely efficacy of the treatment outside the Portuguese climate. Following the Wars, the observations of practitioners like Fergusson who had observed the success of the non-mercurial treatment prompted extensive observation and experiment of non-mercurial treatment in military hospitals in Britain and elsewhere. These trials were supported by McGrigor who corresponded extensively with Edinburgh military surgeon John Thomson about his medical history of the Battle of Waterloo, and also about his proposed publication on the treatment of syphilis.[17] McGrigor strongly encouraged investigation of the treatment and supported the trials being made in various quarters.[18] In 1817 he issued queries to all army surgeons requesting reports on their treatment of the disease and their observations on the non-mercurial treatment. The returns established that of the 4,767 reported cases between 1816 and 1819, 1940 had been treated without mercury. Together he and William Franklin wrote to the surgeons of the army reporting on these results and issuing a cautious endorsement of the therapy.[19] Trials of the approach were also taken up by naval surgeons such as Mr Mortimer the surgeon at Haslar hospital, and observed with interest by his head of department William Burnett.[20] Knowledge of the therapy was not confined to military and naval medical circles. After several years, tracts on the subject addressed to a general medical audience were published by George Guthrie, Thomas Rose and John Thomson.[21] Rose's paper in particular demonstrates the attempts of military practitioners to influence civilian practice. His strong endorsement of the non-mercurial therapy was delivered in a prestigious forum, the Medico Chirurgical Society of London, and printed in the Society's journal. His advocacy of the therapy would have reached many influential ears; unfortunately the requirement that non-mercurially treated patients should remain on absolute bed-rest during the course of their treatment limited the extent to which the practice was taken up by civilian patients.[22] However, more important was the way Rose and his colleagues employed evidence to support their claims. Rose was able to report on a large numbers of trials in military hospitals and regiments.[23] He also detailed personal experience which emphasized both the volume of patients he had treated and his ability to observe them and the effects of their treatment for long periods of time, 'I have during the last two years, treated on the same system more than one hundred and twenty cases, where I have been able to ascertain that my patients were in perfect health for many months afterwards'.[24] In so doing, he was making a claim for the value of military medicine, and mass observation of patients, to a large and influential audience.

It was this promotion of the utility of military experience in combating certain diseases, and the military approach to the investigation of disease, that formed the central plank of the claims military medicine made for an authoritative voice in British medicine in the years following the Wars. These claims were made most strongly in intra-professional disputes that came to be aired in Parliament, and interestingly both centred on diseases that British military practitioners had faced on the Egyptian campaign: ophthalmia and plague.

Parliament and Military Medicine

The efforts of military medical officers to promote their own expertise within the crowded marketplace of post-war Britain, as could be expected, met with some resistance from established practitioners. Several of the debates that resulted were argued and resolved in Parliament, via select committees of inquiry. These inquiries gave the military medical officers their most powerful means of spreading the word of their expertise, and also of convincing some of the most powerful men in the nation of their importance. Parliament was one of the most important tools used by army medical practitioners after the Wars to establish the value of military medicine and its discoveries to British medicine.

Select committee inquiries were used by Parliament to investigate controversial matters or issues on which facts needed to be established before Parliament would consider a motion. Committees could have various powers, including the calling of papers, reports and even the examination of witnesses *viva voce*. They would produce a report that would then be tabled in Parliament with a view to the passing of a motion, or drafting of legislation.[25]

The reports and published evidence of select committees reveal to the historian the issues parliamentarians considered to be important, the types of witness thought to be worth questioning, and the styles of evidence used by witnesses to make their arguments. Thus, they are a rich source of evidence on the interaction between Parliament and military medicine during this period, the status of military practitioners compared with civilian practitioners, the problems of finding an agreed evidentiary model for medical debates and the ways in which Parliament attempted to influence medical practice.

Parliament's Early Involvement

From the beginning of the Wars, and throughout the first part of the nineteenth century, Parliament had engaged in a significant number of inquiries into aspects of medicine, particularly into army medicine and medical issues related to army experience.[26] These early investigations provided military practitioners with an important foundation of politicians well versed in, and sympathetic to, military medical expertise and approaches after the Wars.

The first military medical issues to be considered by select committees of inquiry in the early 1800s were brought to the Commons by medical practitioners themselves. These committees investigated, respectively, Dr Edward Jenner's discovery of vaccine inoculation [vaccination] and Dr Carmichael Smyth's discovery of nitrous fumigation, both in 1802. They were extensive inquiries that called on a large number of medical witnesses. In both cases the medical practitioner in question was petitioning Parliament for public funds as a reward for a useful invention.

The committee investigating Jenner's discovery of vaccine inoculation questioned thirty-six medical witnesses, and six of those were practitioners strongly connected with the military – Sir Gilbert Blane, Mr Francis Knight, Dr Joseph Marshall, Dr John Lind, Mr Thomas Keate and Mr Robert Keate.[27] It is interesting to note that these practitioners were considered of a suitable 'eminence' to give evidence to the committee, however, only Blane, Marshall and Thomas Keate gave evidence related to the effectiveness of vaccination within the forces. Knight and Robert Keate only gave evidence of their opinion of Jenner's originality, and Lind was called specifically to give his opinion on a difficult case.

The evidence of the first three was significantly different to that adduced from the overwhelming majority of medical witnesses to the committee, who had usually testified to their personal experience of vaccination, their opinion of Jenner's originality, and that they had their own children vaccinated.[28] These three witnesses did address those issues, but also discussed their own attempts to introduce vaccination into the service(s) for which they had responsibility, and the efficacy of that measure. In particular, evidence was given by these men on the ability of soldiers and sailors to perform their duties after vaccination (in contrast to smallpox inoculation), whereas the ability of men, women or children to be productive after vaccination was not discussed by any 'civilian' witness. These witnesses also introduced into evidence the positive opinion of vaccination held by senior military leaders under whom they had served. Marshall referred to Admiral Lord Keith and General Sir Ralph Abercrombie.[29] Blane presented testimonials from Lord Keith and General Hutchinson in its favour.[30]

The contribution of military medical officers to this select committee was, admittedly, not overwhelming. However, the quality and content of the military medical submissions does reveal a focus on populations as opposed to individuals, in contrast to the evidence of their civilian colleagues. The only comparable 'civilian' evidence, in this respect, was given by practitioners in charge of large hospitals.[31] It is not possible to determine from the summary form in which the evidence is presented in the report of the committee how extensively the military practitioners were questioned about the productivity of servicemen following vaccination, but the inclusion of the evidence at all suggests that the committee members considered it an important fact. When viewed in combination with the Committee on Nitrous Fumigation, it is clear that parliamentarians had received significant exposure to the distinctive concerns of military medicine, and of 'manpower economy' reasoning, following these two inquiries.[32]

The petitioner in the case of nitrous fumigation was Dr James Carmichael Smyth. Smyth had obtained his MD at Edinburgh University in 1764, in 1788 he was elected a fellow of the Royal College of Physicians, and was elected to the Royal Society in 1799.[33] He had previously been commended by Parliament for his efforts in managing an outbreak of fever among Spanish prisoners in Winchester in 1780, where he had used nitrous fumigation to destroy and prevent contagion.[34] His method was to mix 'pure nitre in powder and concentrated vitriolic acid' in a pipkin that was then carried through the infected area.[35] Fumigation had been used in the fight against contagion throughout history, however Smyth's claim to innovation lay in the ability of patients to remain in the room and breathe during the administration of his fumigation, a circumstance not possible in the common fumigations at the time that used muriatic or sulphuric acids.

In 1795, under the orders of the Lords Commissioners of the Admiralty, he had organized a trial of the nitrous fumigation method on His Majesty's Ship *The Union* at Sheerness.[36] At that time there had been an outbreak of fever that was attributed to the Russian sick that had arrived there. According to the letters and testimonials Smyth presented in his publications, his experiments were a success and were then used widely in the navy, by military surgeons and in prisons.

The select committee investigation into Dr Smyth's discovery of 'Nitrous Fumigation' was initiated by Mr Bragge in the Commons on 25 February 1802. Smyth's petition specifically referred to the usefulness of his discovery to the armed forces.[37] In their report the committee commended not only the practicality of his method 'in situations, such as Ships of War and Transports, where the Removal and Separation of the Sick may be impractical'[38], but also highlighted a consideration they believed to be 'forcibly affecting':

> contagious Fevers have been apt particularly to prevail and make the most dreadful Ravages in Ships of War, or among soldiers, when confined in transports or crowded into Hospitals. It cannot but enhance the Value of the Petitioner's Discovery; and

render the Authentication of its Efficacy a Matter of Satisfaction and Joy, that it provides the Means of arresting the Progress of a most fatal Disease, to which the brave Defenders of their Country must ... be particularly exposed.[39]

They ultimately concluded that the public had benefited from Smyth's discovery, 'especially in the Persons of our brave Soldiers and Sailors'.[40]

Nearly all the witnesses to the committee, both those who appeared in person and those who wrote to it, were connected with either naval or military practice. Their evidence focused strongly not only on the efficacy of Smyth's discovery but also on the practicality of administering it in the less than ideal circumstances of crowded transports and hospitals. Evidence from military practitioners was adduced particularly in relation to the care of Russian sick in the general hospital at Yarmouth in the winter of 1799–1800.[41] A young McGrigor's letters written to Smyth in 1797 were also tendered into evidence.[42] In those letters McGrigor set out his success with the nitrous fumigation against fever and dysentery that afflicted his regiment when stationed in Jersey. He suggested that his might have been the 'first Trial of your excellent Invention in the Army'.[43] McGrigor's letters also set out plainly his perception of military practice as distinct from civilian medicine: 'it has been the means of shewing me a Fact, which, especially in military Practice, I conceive to be of the last [*sic*] Importance'.[44] This distinction had also been made (though less overtly) by other witnesses who distinguished between the use of the fumigation in their military and private practices.

The evidence presented to the committee was not entirely supportive of Dr Smyth's petition. In particular Dr John Lind, surgeon to The Royal Hospital at Haslar, and Dr Thomas Trotter, late physician to the fleet, both objected vehemently to his claims, instead arguing that the widely accepted practices of discipline, separation of the sick and rigorous hygiene were the only sure preventatives against contagion, and that Dr Smyth's fumigation only appeared to be effective because of the time at which it was employed (i.e. at the natural decline of the fever after the aforementioned methods had taken effect).

Lind's arguments against Smyth were based in a defence of his father's (Dr James Lind) measures to prevent contagion, and were ultimately dismissed by the committee because of some inaccuracies.[45] However, Lind's criticism of Smyth's use of statistical tables to prove his success demonstrates the difficulties facing both medical and non-medical experts in inquiries such as this when the efficacy of a particular measure was called into question. Lind's argument was that, despite the apparent success of Smyth's measures as shown in the tables presented in his book, the decrease in morbidity and mortality demonstrated by the tables was actually attributable to the measures that had been put in place before Smyth's methods were implemented and that the tables on their own (or in the context that Smyth had placed them) were misleading. The thrust of Lind's argument was:

while the Nitrous Acid is used only in Combination with Means, which if employed alone, would have been sufficient to have destroyed the Contagion, its Efficacy cannot receive Support from any Result of the combined Means, unless it could have been proved to accelerate them, which is not attempted.[46]

Conversely, Smyth's response to Lind reiterates his support for the evidentiary power of statistics:

> those Regulations of the late Doctor Lind, were either entirely neglected, or executed in so careless and imperfect a Way, as to be totally useless; and that they were so the Returns of the Prison and Hospital for the Six Weeks after he left Winchester, prove in the clearest Manner.[47]

Exchanges such as this, and those which were aired in the ophthalmia inquiry discussed later in this chapter must call into question any perception that the rise of statistics, in the form of naval or military returns, presented an unproblematic way in which to make judgements about medicine and medical efficacy, and certainly did not resolve a failure within the profession to 'achieve a shared framework for interpreting reliable evidence'.[48] While many practitioners and administrators undeniably appreciated this method of record keeping and reporting, the usefulness or ways of using those records in actual debate had not been established and many, like Lind, instinctively grasped the meaninglessness of statistics divorced from the circumstances in which they were produced.

Trotter's antagonism to Smyth's method was based in a strong philosophical objection to the use of fumigation *per se*. In his evidence he stridently objected to the practice of fumigation that he insinuated was supported only by mystery, the occult, superstition and 'relics of exorcism'.[49] Trotter is well known for his commitment to achieving health through discipline, the enlistment of officers in hygienic measures and the occupation of the mind.[50] His evidence against fumigation was entirely consistent with his philosophy. Fumigation only appeared to work, he argued, because it was inevitably used at the same time as those other methods of combating disease. Moreover, he warned that fumigation gave a false sense of security, which could undermine the practice of the necessary discipline and hygiene that in reality prevented contagion.

The more interesting argument offered by Trotter was his analysis of Smyth's case for fumigation which Trotter labelled 'assertion instead of proof', and which essentially accused Smyth of relying on *post hoc ergo propter hoc* reasoning.[51] What Trotter required for proof he said, was reasoning based in theory and accepted principles, not speculation and conjecture. Trotter's evidence demonstrates the complexities of the divisions within the medical profession regarding the probative value of certain types of proof: his thoroughly modern, military medical officer-like support for preventative measures and the importance of support from officers in their implementation is expressed at the same time as his much more 'establishment' view that deduction from 'mere observation', even in large volume, should not be enough to change accepted medical views, and only innovations which could be explained by new discoveries in the history of the disease or the explained specific nature of the medicine were acceptable.[52]

The committee gave extensive consideration to Trotter's allegations, investigating in detail the surgeon's journals on the ships on which Trotter submitted a fever had been defeated without the use of nitrous acid. They found some inaccuracies in his evidence regarding practices on various ships, and had evidence presented from an apothecary and a chemist that ostensibly contradicted his views about the nitrous acid. Ultimately, the committee tacitly endorsed Smyth's rebuttal that, in fact, it was Trotter who was making the 'assertions'.[53] It does appear that the committee were not prepared, or possibly able, to engage with the theoretical position presented by Trotter, and it is possible that ultimately evidence they were able to understand, 'experiential' evidence, carried more weight with them.

The committee's report was presented to the Commons by Mr Bankes on 10 June 1802 [54] and on 24 June 1802 the House resolved *nemine contradicente* that Smyth's discovery had:

> already been attended with the most beneficial effects, especially in His Majesty's Naval and Military Hospitals ... it may justly be expected to be hereafter productive of the most extensive advantages, particularly to his Majesty's fleets and armies

The House recommended an award of £5,000.[55]

These two committees demonstrate that medical issues were being considered by Parliament early in the Wars, and that the military medical voice at those investigations was given significant weight. They also demonstrate that modes of persuasion beginning to be used by military practitioners, such as 'manpower economy' arguments and statistical evidence, were aired in Parliament, albeit with varying levels of success. Importantly, ultimately it was the parliamentarians who decided the value of these discoveries, their newness and what they were worth. This was particularly important in cases, such as the latter, when questions of 'medical expertise' were raised, and the value of various types of evidence brought to the attention of the committee.

Military medical issues were brought to the attention of Parliament again soon after the conclusion of the two inquiries just considered, in the form of the Commissioners of Military Enquiry's investigation of the AMD and their 'Fifth Report' which were discussed in Chapter 2. As already noted, that inquiry went directly to the division between civilian and military medicine which developed during the Wars, and to how Parliament involved itself in that debate. The patterns it set in train are directly relevant to the way in which medical professionals used select committees later in the period. Many of these issues were rehearsed again in the Walcheren inquiry a few years later.

As has been shown, the debates between the military and civilian branches of the medical profession were related to differences in the educational models each branch generally pursued. Many of the 'new' types of evidence being advanced by military practitioners had grown out of the ways in which they were required to manage and report on their practice. Parliamentarians were exposed to another dose of this debate in one of the most important developments in the regulation of medical education in Britain immediately following the Wars, the Apothecaries Act of 1815. The genesis and operation of this Act has been extensively researched by Irvine Loudon in his seminal work on the general practitioner.[56] However, one particular aspect of that Act that is regularly mentioned, but which remains under-researched, is the attempt to have army and navy surgeons exempted from its operation in relation to educational prerequisites and examination required for certification.

The initial bill included a clause excluding persons acting or having acted as full surgeon or apothecary in the army or navy from examination under the Act, however it was removed after the bill was sent to the Act of Parliament Committee of the Society of Apothecaries and no such exclusion was legislated until 1825.[57] That committee, which was not a parliamentary committee, had received a letter from the College of Physicians in January 1814 commenting on the then proposed bill and requiring 'that all persons who have acted in any Department of the Army or Navy as Medical Practitioners should not thence derive any authority to practice unless examined by the constituted bodies'.[58] The non-inclusion of the army and navy surgeons' exemption caused problems for the examiners under the Act almost as soon as it was passed, because many army and navy surgeons had not served a five-year apprenticeship as required by the legislation. The examiners requested advice from counsel on the matter, asking what to do regarding army and navy surgeons 'whose qualifications are in many instances superior to those of others'.[59] The position of the military surgeons remained unclear and further opinions from counsel were sought and applications to Parliament to resolve the matter considered.[60] Many of the arguments put to counsel for consideration were based on the notion that the education of army and navy surgeons was equal, and probably superior to, that of a 'regular' candidate for examination who had served the requisite time in an apprenticeship. In April 1816 the AMB requested a conference with the Principal Officers of the Company of Apothecaries, or the Court of Examiners.[61] At that meeting the chairman of the committee told the AMB 'that the Society had no intention whatever of taking any measures to prevent such surgeons of the Army whose warrants bear date previously from practicing as Apothecaries'.[62] The AMB then required the apothecaries to 'give some public testimony' of that intention, and

accordingly the Committee passed a resolution to that effect.[63] In May that year
it was proposed to make an application to Parliament to amend the *Apothecaries
Act* to enable surgeons of the army and navy of certain years' standing to practice
without certificate, and to that end members of the Committee sought a meeting with Lord Palmerston who apparently gave his wholehearted support to the
measure.[64] It does not appear that any such amendment was actually legislated;
however the position of the army and navy surgeons may have been considered
settled by the resolution of the committee.

Lord Palmerston was only one of several parliamentarians who were involved
in the creation and administration of the Apothecaries Act. However, it is not
clear whether any of the wrangling over the position of military surgeons, or the
College of Physician's opposition to their exemption under the Act came directly
to the attention of a wider parliamentary audience. What is clear is that parliamentarians such as Lord Palmerston were approached to help resolve the matter;
further establishing the impression that Parliament was seen by many practitioners as a forum for deciding medical debates. It is also clear from the failure of
military surgeons to keep the exclusion in the initial bill, that by the end of the
Wars, army and navy surgeons did not feel that they had the necessary authority and backing to completely convince Parliament that the education they had
received and their experience on-the-field were examination enough to place
them ahead of their civilian counterparts who had to be examined under the Act.

After the Wars military practitioners continued to bring medical debates to
Parliament in their efforts to secure a competitive advantage over their civilian
counterparts. The arguments that were voiced by the two sides were grounded
in the different educational models each branch generally pursued. Many of the
'new' types of evidence being advanced by military practitioners had grown out
of the ways in which they were required to manage and report on their practice.
In these inquiries the questions of what type of medical experience, and what
medical paradigm, would be considered best was brought squarely to the attention of a Parliament that had been schooled throughout the Wars in the value of
military medicine.

Parliament and Plague

Military medical officers had gained much experience in dealing with and preventing the spread of plague during the Egyptian campaign, and in subsequent
outbreaks in the Mediterranean. The parliamentary inquiry into the contagiousness of the plague held in 1819 gave them the opportunity to promote their
expertise and attempt to influence national policy on the question of whether
plague should be treated as a contagious disease

This inquiry was precipitated by the manoeuvring of a very politically active medical practitioner, Charles Maclean.[65] Maclean had gained most of his medical experience in the tropics with the East India Company, and had also enlisted as an army medical officer in 1804. Unfortunately, MacLean fell foul of Lucas Pepy's AMB, owing to his lack of an Oxbridge education. While he had made strenuous efforts to be promoted when serving with the army in the years 1804–5, he believed that he had been denied that opportunity by the AMB while operating under Pepys' 'civilian friendly' recruitment policy. He resigned from the army in 1805, but like other prominent army medical officers, Maclean championed the value of medical experience gained overseas, and experience over theory in general.

Maclean believed that almost no diseases were contagious. He was particularly adamant in this respect about the plague.[66] Maclean had been trying to persuade the medical profession of his 'theory of epidemic disease' and non-contagion since the turn of the century, but had been spectacularly unsuccessful. Eventually he gave up trying to persuade the medical profession and turned his attention to the public and to Parliament, perhaps thinking that if he could persuade them, his theory would become the dominant one.[67]

He did this in several different ways. First, Maclean was no stranger to publications in newspapers and journals that he continued to pursue. Secondly, he made his 'theory of epidemic disease' more exciting by adding some elements sure to catch the attention of politicians, businessmen and the public: an attack on the Catholic Church and the economic cost of quarantine. Importantly, for the purposes of this discussion, he also cultivated politically powerful patrons and agitated to have the issue debated in Parliament.

Since 1813, Maclean had been cultivating the patronage of the Duke of Kent, the Levant Company, Lord Grenville and the East India Company.[68] They supported him in an expedition to the Levant to research the plague in late 1815. *Results of an Investigation Regarding Epidemic and Pestilential Diseases*, the two-volume account of his research there, is usually seen as the catalyst for the 1819 parliamentary inquiry.[69] Lord Grenville presented *Results* to the Levant Company Court who, in turn, asked Grenville to present it on their behalf to the Prince Regent and request an inquiry.[70]

In February 1819, Sir John Jackson, a director of the East India Company, rose in the Commons to call for a select committee to consider the 'Validity of the Doctrine of Contagion in the Plague'. He was supported by Mr Robinson, treasurer of the navy and member of the Board of Trade.[71] The inquiry that followed is particularly interesting in the context of this chapter, not because of the complex opinions that were aired about the nature of contagion, but because the way in which Maclean directed the debate required practitioners to address the question of what type of evidence should be probative, theory or experience.

While the committee concluded that there was no evidence to support a change to the 'received doctrine of contagion', these findings do not accurately represent the proceedings of the committee, which thoroughly investigated the opinion of nearly every witness on the quarantine laws and found that the great majority supported their amendment. Sir John Jackson chaired the inquiry and was clearly persuaded by the argument of the anticontagionists.[72] He refused to sign the contagionist report of the committee and spoke against it in Parliament.[73] Of the nineteen medical practitioners examined by the committee, nine had served with the army or navy. Practitioners were specifically questioned as to whether their knowledge of the plague came from personal experience or the accounts of others.

The proceedings directly addressed the question of whether non-medically trained politicians could determine whether a disease was contagious, and the opinions of Maclean and other practitioners specifically fought on the issue. Maclean was given the floor in his second address to the committee and definitively stated, 'In conclusion, I may observe, that the question of contagion in epidemic diseases, as acknowledged even by its advocates, *is entirely one of fact, not of physic*, of which all persons of a liberal education are as competent to judge as physicians'.[74] Such arguments directly undercut the importance of medical texts and theory.

A further committee in 1824 considered the effect of quarantine on the foreign trade of Britain but not the question of contagion, which was considered settled by the 1819 report.[75] Medical witnesses were consulted by this committee, but only contagionists, as the opinion of anticontagionists on quarantine regulations was considered a foregone conclusion. The committee concluded that the quarantine system was too onerous and recommended that the length of quarantine be reduced and penalties for contravention made less harsh. Debates on the successful Quarantine Laws Bill in Parliament in the following year were accompanied by a petition from Maclean introduced into Parliament by John Smith.[76] Smith gave strong support to Maclean and advocated the view that 'the question, as to its contagious or non-contagious quality, was not so much a question of science as a question of fact, on which any man who was in the habit of weighing testimony, was qualified to decide'.[77]

However, the parliamentary forum for medical debate was not approved of by many practitioners, who felt that non-medics would only be able to appreciate experience-based evidence and not the finer points of medical learning and theory that they believed were essential. The eminent naval physician Sir Gilbert Blane was a witness to both committees. He was deeply concerned by Maclean's attack on the profession stating that it had exposed the 'dignity of the profession' to 'the sneers of the extra-professional part of the community'.[78] He feared that division within the profession would cause public health authorities to 'ask the assistance of some members of the bench or the bar accustomed to weigh evidence, and investigate facts, or even of such plain men as compose juries, than medical men, having so much reason to suspect that our minds are warped by prejudice'.[79]

The participants in this debate were conscious of the evidentiary problems with which they struggled, referring to 'the unsettled nature of the laws of evidence in regard to medical inquiries',[80] and the need to establish meaningful ground on which to engage in a conflict of ideas. The debates over the type of evidence presented to the committee mirror those encountered in the select committee inquiries considered earlier in this chapter. The essential point being that according a higher value to 'experience'-based evidence placed the educational model of men like the military medical officer above those who had been traditionally educated.

The relevance of overseas medical innovation and army practice to this debate was grasped by Maclean, who argued that the 'establishment's' myopic view of medicine was obstructing the adoption of practices developed by the experimental approach fostered in the Scottish universities, the military and overseas.[81] In addition, Maclean's influence on the direction of contagion debates, and his passionate support for the empirical/experimental approach, ensured that this issue was embedded in the considerations of the antagonists. The statements of witnesses to the inquiries and the writings of eminent physicians demonstrated a struggle on both sides of the debate to establish what type of evidence would be probative in not only this, but all medical debates, and what type of witness would be considered competent to give it.

Predictably, the Royal College of Physicians maintained most strongly the value of ancient texts, asserting in their report to Parliament on Maclean's *Results* that considerable evidence would be required to counterbalance the 'weight of ages'.[82] However, this position was undermined by some 'establishment' practitioners who, while not rejecting the importance of theory, argued for the importance of experience. In his evidence to the 1824 inquiry, Augustus Bozzi Granville, MD, made a clear statement that he wanted his evidence to be confined to 'practical, not theoretical' matters. He believed that the 'theoretical' evidence given to the 1819 inquiry had done more harm than good and implied that the evidence of witnesses who 'had never seen the plague ... and spoke merely from theoretical views' could lead to 'no useful conclusion'.[83] Even Sir Gilbert Blane, when considering the question, concluded that the two modes of reasoning should be given equal weight.[84]

This conflict between two probative systems was evident to the layperson, and in the 1819 inquiry Jackson directly asked Dr William Gladstone, surgeon to the naval asylum at Greenwich, whether he would 'rather be governed by modern facts' or 'historical reports?'[85]

Contagion and quarantine were perceived to be very important to the national interest and the most frequent complaint in the press was dissatisfaction with the quality of argument from all parties. The consensus was that nearly all medical practitioners, particularly Maclean, approached the question full of prejudice.[86] The parliamentary inquiries were not considered to have decided the question and calls were made for *impartial* investigation.[87] In Parliament, John Smith argued for the appointment of a commission 'consisting of medical practitioners partly, and partly of men of general science and experience, charged to collect and examine into, and observe facts connected with the propagation of the plague'.[88]

The debates aired during the contagion inquiry threw into sharp relief the evidentiary struggle between two paradigms, the importance of which to military medical officers lay in the experiential model valuing more highly the observations of practitioners who had personally observed and treated a disease. Such a value system would automatically count more highly the opinions of practitioners who had served overseas where those diseases were more prevalent. The gradual acceptance of this form of evidence is demonstrated by statements such as that of Mr Hume who stated in a parliamentary debate that he 'would certainly prefer the opinions of those who had visited the countries in which the plague occasionally showed itself'.[89]

Parliament and Egyptian Ophthalmia

Competition between military and civilian practitioners after the Wars was most violently debated on the question of Egyptian ophthalmia. As shown in Chapter 3, the disease raged in British regiments long after the conclusion of the Egyptian campaign in 1801. In the decade following 1809 it produced a vast number of invalids and pensioners over which military and civilian practitioners, backed by their political patrons, engaged in a bitter dispute for the right to treat.

The civilian protagonist at the centre of this dispute was Sir William Adams.[90] Adams had trained under John Cunningham Saunders at The London Infirmary for curing diseases of the eye in Charterhouse Square. In 1807, he had established his own practice in Exeter, where he helped to establish the West of England Infirmary for curing eye disease. He claimed marvellous success in the treatment of gutta serena and cataracts and also to have developed a procedure to treat the third stage of the Egyptian ophthalmia, which involved the repeated removal of granulations on the palpabrae with a scalpel. Saunders had also employed this technique using scissors. Adams treated the inflammatory stages of the disease with extensive vomits.

Adams became very successful and was made surgeon and oculist-extraordinary to the Prince Regent and to the dukes of Kent and Sussex, and he was knighted in 1814. He had other powerful patrons, the commander in chief, Sir David Dundas, and the secretary at war, Lord Palmerston. In 1817, he was given the charge of an ophthalmic hospital in Regents Park, and set up by his patrons in opposition to army medical officers who claimed superior skills in the treatment of the Egyptian ophthalmia. Adams's elevation incurred the particular ire of the AMB and McGrigor, who had become its director general in 1815. Their dispute over the 'territory of ophthalmia' was made known to the public through the publication of various pamphlets and reports by each side, through the medical press, a select committee inquiry, and was finally debated in Parliament.

Adams's side of the story is set out in detail in several documents; his letter to the directors of the Greenwich Hospital,[91] a report of the directors of Greenwich Hospital,[92] and another published anonymously in 1821.[93]

The latter of those documents states that Adams was first noticed in 1810 by General Thewles, the commander of the Western District who informed Sir David Dundas of Adams's successes. This pamphlet suggests that Dundas took a particular interest in Adams, to whom he was introduced in 1810, and that he initiated a trial of Adams's practice, intending to give him small number of ophthalmic patients so that he could 'prove on them his practice'.[94] However, the pamphleteer alleges that the AMB was consulted about this trial and created obstacles that prevented the trial from going ahead. Adams was given another opportunity to prove himself when, in 1811, the adjutant general called him to the Horse Guards and asked him about his treatment for the ophthalmia. The adjutant general then assured Adams of the support of the commander-in-chief, the AMB, and of letters expressing the support of his Royal Highness.

The anonymous *Facts and Documents* goes on to recount that the adjutant general ordered the then director general of the AMB, Dr Weir, to provide a sergeant and six patients to Adams. The men were to be told that they would get discharges if their sight was restored. However, from the first interview in 1812 the AMD was 'decidedly hostile' and tried to 'frustrate his views and counteract his efforts'. These allegations against the AMB were supported by the inclusion of a letter issued by the adjutant general to the director general of the AMB on 2 December 1812. In that letter the director general was ordered to give Adams the patients and communicate to Adams their history:

> in order that a point so essentially involving, not only the health of individuals, but the efficiency of the army at large, may be decided in the only satisfactory way, by a fair experiment of the efficacy of Mr. Adam's mode of treatment.[95]

It appears that following this letter Adams made several experiments on pensioners but army practitioners contested the results of those experiments.

In their publication, the directors of Greenwich Hospital tell how Adams also examined the blind pensioners at Greenwich Hospital and selected twenty for operation 'consisting of Cataracts, Closed Pupils, and the Egyptian Ophthalmia'. The medical officers of the hospital were directed to attend the operations, give assistance and report to the directors.[96] The operations were recorded an astounding success by the hospital physician, surgeon, and apothcary:

> In addition to the gratifying contents of the second Report, we think it our duty to state, for the information of the Board, that Mr. Adams has discovered a mode of curing the Egyptian Ophthalmia, which has been successfully practiced upon several of the Pensioners, some of whom had been blind for three or four years, and given up as incurable by the most eminent Oculists then in London. The communication that this destructive and hitherto intractable Disease admits of cure we conceive will be gladly received by the Board, and the promulgation by Mr Adams of this important discovery be considered as a great *national desideratum*.[97]

On reading this report the directors convened a special meeting to 'examine and individually interrogate' Adams's patients. They found the reports of the physician, surgeon and apothecary to be accurately detailed and decided to give publicity to the reports and proceedings 'on a subject so interesting to humanity'.[98]

Unfortunately for Adams, the hostility of the AMB continued. His anonymous supporter records that in 1813, the commander-in-chief gave directions that an inquiry into Adams's practice

> should be taken entirely out of the hands of *Army Practitioners* (who at *that time*, most pertinaciously denied its efficacy), and that it should be placed in those of the following eminent *Civilian Practitioners*: Sir Henry Halford, Bart., Dr. Baillie, Sir Everard Home, Bart., H. Cline, Esq., Astley Cooper, Esq. and J Abernethy, Esq.[99]

Following favourable reports from those gentlemen, Adams understood that it was the intention of His Royal Highness and the secretary of state for the Home Department and of the secretary at war to adopt his plan to establish a hospital for the treatment of ophthalmic disorders. According to this record, those plans were thwarted by McGrigor, who had been promoted to the director generalship of the AMB in June 1815. The report makes the serious allegation that on 4 July 1815, McGrigor wrote to the adjutant general regarding the Egyptian ophthalmia stating:

> there now remain but a few cases in the neighbourhood of Plymouth, and I trust that this disorder will soon be eradicated from the army ... the discoveries of late years relating to it, and other Disease of the Eye, *being* now *very generally promulgated* and the attention of *some medical officers of the army being* now *directed to those diseases*, I have no doubt but that from the service *I can select* officers perfectly equal to the cure of those diseases, where a cure can be effected ... the establishment proposed by Sir. W. Adams is by no means required, as its objects can be obtained without incurring any further expense.[100]

Despite McGrigor's claims, the secretary at war called for the returns of ophthalmic diseases treated in the army hospitals since 1810. They showed, contrary to McGrigor's figures, that the malady was extensively prevailing. McGrigor continued to send letters to the secretary at war asserting that the ophthalmia had 'ceased to prevail in the British Army for several years'. The final claim against McGrigor in this document is that in 1816, he used all his influence to form an eye infirmary placing 'an Army Surgeon, a personal friend of the Director General ... at the head of this institution'.[101]

The army surgeon and personal friend of McGrigor referred to was Dr John Vetch. Vetch and Adams turned to the press to assert their respective claims to superiority. In 1817, Adams published his *Letter*, and in the following year Vetch published a pamphlet of observations on Adams's treatment.[102] Adams believed he was the victim of a conspiracy of army medical officers and purported to be defending himself against attacks made on his 'honor and integrity'. The medical grounds on which Vetch and Adams actually engaged were the treatment of the inflammatory stages of the disease, Vetch using the bleeding treatment and Adams using vomits, and the originality of Adams's treatment of the third stage of the disease. The *Edinburgh Medical and Surgical Journal* weighed in on the debate and declared Vetch the winner. The editor also made strong statements condemning the 'unfair' advantage Adams had been given by his patrons, 'over the regular army surgeons', who it was clearly implied were being poorly rewarded for their brave service during the Wars.[103] In 1817, The secretary at war had decided to found an ophthalmic hospital and place Adams at its head. Eventually, the post of ophthalmic surgeon to the army was also created for him, at a salary of £1,500, which Courtney understates 'greatly offended the military surgeons'.[104]

Vetch claimed to have successfully treated more than 3,000 cases and challenged the 'grounds on which Sir Wm Adams has advanced pretensions to the discovery of "those new and successful methods of treating the disease", which have been announced to the army, in the circular letter of the Rt Hon. The Secretary at War dated August 1817.' Vetch criticized Adams's use of violent vomiting in early stage of disease, and suggested that he would never have used that treatment if he had seen a real case of Egyptian ophthalmia. Vetch thought that Adams's conclusions must have been based on a form of the disease mainly seen in children when crowded together. Or that his experience had been confined to the military asylum 'where the age or sex of the patients prevented it ever acquiring the excessive violence which it assumed in the army', thus challenging his competence to treat soldiers.[105]

Vetch claimed that his experience with the Egyptian ophthalmia in the army had demonstrated to him (and he had written about) the importance of the granular surface of the linings of the palpebrae, and that he had discovered the means to restore the membrane to its healthy condition before he ever could have read Saunders, i.e. before Adams was using the treatment.[106] He also argued that the method used by Adams to fix the palpabrae was counter-productive and that 'the treatment I adopted in the disease, does not require the aid of an operation in one case out of fifty'.[107] He further supported his claim to first calling the attention of the AMB to the importance of restoring the healthy state of the palpebral linings previous to the discharge of the patients by citing a letter from David Dundas dated 9 November 1809, which cleared him of allowing patients to malinger by keeping them until the linings were clear.[108]

The dispute over the priority of discovery regarding the palpabrael linings was continued by Adams who published a reply to Vetch.[109] His claims are those to be expected, and he criticized in particular the extensive bleeding used by Vetch, thereby criticizing the 'gospel' practice amongst military practitioners.[110]

The existence of two institutions for the treatment of the ophthalmic pensioners soon came to the attention of a budget-conscious Parliament, and on 11 May 1819, Mr J. P. Grant rose to ask why

> the ophthalmia having prevailed to a considerable extent in our army, an hospital had, during the war, been established at Bognor for the cure of that disorder; great cures of it had been effected; and the disease was found of late years to have happily abated in the army. Notwithstanding this, in a time of peace, and at a moment when public economy was so much talked of, not only a new establishment was formed, but a gentleman (Sir W. Adams) was placed at the head of it, who had never been in the army; and who had therefore no claim to military patronage ... and who, though he was not even now in the army was placed over the heads of many eminent men who had devoted their lives to the service of their country[111]

Grant set out an argument very similar to that advanced in Vetch's works, stressing the priority of army medical officers in the treatment of this disease. He called for an inquiry into the establishment of the second institution and for all the papers relating to its establishment.

Lord Palmerston responded to Grant's motion and used the opportunity to give his version of the history of the establishment of Adams's ophthalmic hospital. He suggested that Grant had received most of his information from Dr Vetch 'who, he understood, had been of opinion that he ought to have been made the superintendent of the new establishment, instead of Sir W. Adams'.[112] Palmerston went on to state that the army medical practitioners had been so opposed to Adams and his mode of treatment, even after the report from eminent practitioners in 1814, that 'it was useless to think of associating Sir W. Adams with them; and the only way of rendering his system generally available was to place himself at the head of the establishment'.[113] Palmerston also introduced to the House his personal observations of the patients in Adams's hospital, and invited the members to go there and judge for themselves. Finally, to prove the

hostility of the medical men of the army, Palmerston read to the House an inter-
cepted letter that appeared to prove a conspiracy in which an army practitioner
connived to get Adams's patients drunk and thus induce a relapse of the disease
before an inspection. Palmerston did not, however, consent to the production of
the papers because they would 'not contribute to real information, or lead to useful discussion'.[114] The motion was debated but finally it was negatived without
any call for a division.[115]

In response to Palmerston's claim that the papers did not need to be produced,
Vetch wrote him a public letter.[116] In that letter he stressed the importance of
army medical experience to treat soldiers. This superiority of army practitioners
was not a negative reflection on Adams, but arose instead 'from the superior experience of the Medical Officers of the Army in these diseases'.[117] Vetch supported
this claim by stating that army practitioners could devote all their time to the ophthalmia spreading through the forces whereas the civil oculist was more diversely
occupied. Vetch also drew attention to the high number of desertions that he
claimed Adams caused because he did not understand the character of soldiers.

Vetch also made reference to the initial trial undertaken by Adams, and
to the conflicting evaluations of that trial. Vetch expressed particular outrage
at Palmerston's reasons for suppressing a report critical of Adams's practice,
opposing Palmerston's view that it was 'dictated by a spirit of professional jeal-
ousy and hostile combination against Sir William Adams'. Furthermore, Vetch
did not agree 'that your Lordship's own testimony, and the statement given by
Sir William Adams himself, render further evidence not only unnecessary, but
inadmissible'.[118] To this end, Vetch included the text of a report made by Dr Benjamin Moseley, physician to Chelsea Hospital, Thomas Keate, Esq. chairman to
the College of Surgeons and the late surgeon-general to the army, and William
North, Esq., dated 17 March 1818. This report found that of sixty-four Scottish
pensioners selected by Adams for treatment thirty were still unfit and the thirty-
four 'supposed' to have been cured, had not been and were very liable to relapses.
The report recommended waiting before sending the 2–3,000 more pensioners
for treatment.[119] Vetch also included two similar letters dated 29 April 1818 and
24 August 1818. The second of these concluded:

> hence it should seem to us, that it were well, as we have already observed, to let these
> men remain quietly at their homes, rather than subject them to the inconveniences
> of long marches, and sea voyages, in addition to the uncertainty of unusual treatment
> and hazardous experiments.[120]

Finally, on 6 March 1821 it was moved in Parliament that a committee of inquiry
be established to give Adams 'an opportunity of vindicating his reputation, and
proving the merits of the institution over which he presided'. The motion was
backed by supporters of Adams and others who knew medical gentlemen 'at var-

iance' with Adams and wanted to get to the bottom of the matter.[121] The motion was carried and in 1821 the committee issued its report.[122] Its findings were generally supportive of Adams's practice, although it questioned his discovery of the palpabrael cure, suggesting instead that he had merely revived something that had been known since antiquity. The commissioners also stated that they were 'induced to think very highly' of the 'knowledge and skill of Dr. Vetch'. They found that, 'the objects of the Establishment, having now been attained', there did not appear to be 'any public inconvenience [that] would now arise from its discontinuance'. Such aims included diffusion of the successful techniques generally among the surgeons of the army and establishing the best mode of treating the chronic, or third stage, of the disorder. They also recommended that Adams be awarded £4,000 for his services to the public. That award was contested in Parliament by Mr H. G. Bennet who 'was one of those who thought that not a penny of the public money should be given to that gentleman'.[123] Lord Palmerston defended the claim and the full £4,000 was paid to Adams.

In the course of this debate, Adams had made overt claims of McGrigor's untruthfulness, and those claims had been (less overtly) repeated by Lord Palmerston. Unusually, McGrigor, who was given to strident rebuttals of any such allegation made against him, did not issue any statement denying that he had lied to his superiors about the extent of the ophthalmia. In 1819, however, McGrigor had published a document that set out his opinion of Adams and strongly asserted the superiority of army practitioners for the treatment of this disorder. With William Franklin, McGrigor argued that Adams was no better than many civil and army oculists and in the treatment of Egyptian ophthalmia he was worse than army medical officers because he did not have their experience. McGrigor further explained that Adams's lack of understanding was not only medical but also cultural in that he did not understand soldiers' dislike of submitting to operations at the judgement of only one person, and that in army practice (under the orders of the commander-in-chief) there was always, in such cases, a consultation. McGrigor and Franklin further claimed that as result of Adams's practice there had been many desertions. To support their argument they attached medical reports unfavourable to Adams.[124] In addition, it appears that the case conducted by the AMB against Adams before the select committee had been vitriolic. Mr J. Dawson commented on the proceedings before the committee, defending the non-production of the papers to Parliament, stating:

> The quarrels between nations and empires were never carried on with half the ferocity which distinguished the quarrels of bigots and authors. But of all the quarrels that had ever occurred between men of science, there was not one that displayed more ill feeling than that which distinguished the dispute between the Medical Board and Sir William Adams.[125]

The *Edinburgh Medical and Surgical Journal* reviewed the pamphlets that had been produced by Adams and the AMB after the establishment of Adam's hospital. The editor was deeply critical of Adams's lack of military experience, contrasting him with McGrigor, 'the man who had attended the Indian Army across the Desert to Egypt; – who had studied ophthalmia in its cradle'.[126] He also made a scathing assessment of the proceedings before Parliament:

> These proceedings will remain a salutary lesson to those who, filching from the fair fame of others, may hereafter submit their illusory claims to the tribunal of the public; while they may tend in some degree to moderate the self-complacency of non-professional men, who conceive themselves intuitively competent to decide on grave professional subjects.[127]

The claim within this statement, that parliamentarians were not qualified to be the arbiters of medical debates, was raised by many concerned practitioners during this period, especially during the deliberations of the select committee on the contagiousness of the plague. The fact remained, however, that Parliament was, by this time, deeply involved in medical debates, and had been embroiled in those relating to the military medical profession for over twenty years. The pamphlets published by the central players in this debate make clear that the committee was faced with a civilian versus military practitioner dispute that was very marked, very open and very bitter. It was also presented with varying types of medical evidence, not the least of which was statistical tables and refutations of those tables. It was even confronted with different assertions of who was cured and who was not. It is perhaps not surprising, in such circumstances, that members of the House chose to instead assert their own ability to assess medical practices and decide between two competing ones.

The make-up of the select committee in this instance is worth noting, as it comprised many very senior and influential men, several of whom requested to join the committee after it had initially been formed.[128] Most importantly, in the debates in Parliament it is clear that the medical protagonists had procured powerful political patrons who felt very passionately about the issue themselves. It seems clear that the participants on both sides of the debate were keen for the issue to be taken to Parliament, and also that they supplemented their efforts in that direction with appeals to the public through written works. These tactics of 'exciting interest' in their cause bear great similarity to those of the Benthamites identified by Finer, and demonstrate that the sophistication of the tactics used by military medical practitioners to disseminate the value of their expertise throughout British society.[129]

Conclusion

McGrigor's appointment to the head of the AMD meant that he was placed at the centre of a global network of military medical officers, and expanded the 'hub' role he had adopted throughout his medical career. It allowed him to attempt to adopt a role in the field of medicine similar to that which had been held by Sir Joseph Banks in the natural sciences.[130] A review of his correspondence in the first few years after the Wars demonstrates that his efforts to promote the medical discoveries of the Wars and of practitioners serving in distant climates were strenuous. The question of whether he continued to pursue a similar model of inquiry and dissemination throughout the rest of his career warrants further research.

Demobilization thrust a large number of ex-military medical officers upon the British medical marketplace. Many of these men were successful in establishing civilian careers and in placing themselves in hospital positions where they were able to influence the development of young doctors and the expectations of patients. They took with them not only therapeutics and medical practices that had been developed and honed during the Wars, but also an approach to the doctor–patient relationship that were all closely allied with the hospital medicine that gradually came to dominate British medicine over the next century. Through the practice of their medicine in the civilian sphere, military medical practitioners helped to pave the way for this transition.

More deliberately, military medical officers promoted the value of their experience in Parliament. This was especially the case in issues relating to divisions between the military and civilian arms of the medical profession, and in cases where an intra-professional resolution was not possible because of a lack of an agreed probative basis for engaging in medical debate. Medical practitioners supplemented their appeals to Parliament with pamphlets addressed to the public, and at the same time it is clear that medical practitioners believed it was important to cultivate political patrons, and they did so assiduously. These patrons appear to have become significantly interested in the medical perspectives they championed and the involvement of men such as Viscount Palmerston and Lord Grenville in medicine during this period also warrants further research.

The effect of this increased parliamentary attention to medical matters was inevitably that the medical debates raised in Parliament were resolved in Parliament, not by medical practitioners themselves. It also appears that many parliamentarians considered themselves eminently qualified to make such determinations, and that they were supported in that conclusion by some medical practitioners who espoused the availability of medical knowledge to all. Although many practitioners continued to claim the exclusivity of knowledge and authority, this authority was ceded, in part, to parliamentarians the moment the question was taken up by them. The availability of knowledge was closely linked to the constitution of that knowledge, and accordingly medical practitioners presented different ways of proving medical facts to Parliament. The types of evidence that appear to have been favoured in the parliamentary forum were those grounded in personal observation and experience. Thus the educational model promoted by military medical officers was tacitly endorsed. The ability of Parliament to promote one type of medical practice or opinion over another was perceived by medical practitioners who exploited the potential thus presented.

Ultimately the engagement of military medical officers with Parliament diminished in part any claim they may have had to exclusivity of medical knowledge, but endorsed a model of medical expertise most beneficial to that group of practitioners.

CONCLUSION

The conquest of disease has long been considered vital to the expansion of the British Empire. Conversely, encounters with new disease environments in India, the West Indies and the Americas have been identified as catalysts for evolutions in the way disease, therapeutics and the British constitution were understood. One of the most significant of these periods of change was the early nineteenth century. This study has endeavoured to bridge the gap between histories establishing the effects of foreign service and the experience of war on British medical practitioners, and studies investigating the transition from older forms of knowledge, to 'hospital' or empirically-based medicine. With the exception of a handful of recently published works, the contribution of British army medical officers of the French Revolutionary and Napoleonic Wars to that process has not been explored, despite the fact that those practitioners formed a significant proportion of the British medical community and were likely to have had some influence on the development of medical theory and practice.

Such recently published works have exploded traditional military medical histories that dismissed these practitioners as ill-educated butchers purveying a medicine based on misguided science. The successes of disease prevention during this period have also been shown to have been based on more than a fortuitous alignment of circumstance. Additionally, historians have begun to illuminate the ways in which new forms of medical evidence and reporting were constructed by these practitioners. It has also been established that they did all these things within a context in which it was necessary to cultivate military or political patronage in order to succeed.

To understand the effect of the Wars on British medicine more generally it was essential to properly investigate how their military experience changed the medical and professional philosophies of army medical officers. This study has sought to establish these effects by considering the accounts of their service given by medical practitioners of the Wars: their official and personal letters, diaries, published writings and the arguments they used during official investigations. In so doing, the myriad and often vitriolic disputes within the medical service, between medical and civilian practitioners, medical practitioners and army officers, and those in which politicians became involved, were uncovered – and they have been the central focus of this work. In analysing such disputes the medical practitioners' modes of rhetoric, motivations and strategies for recruiting allies have been closely examined. It has been concluded that the vast majority of these debates were, at their core, about the type of knowledge which should be considered probative in medical debates, and that for many reasons military medical practitioners were striving to assert the authority of observationally-based, empirical medicine which shared many of the characteristics of what has been identified by other historians as hospital medicine.

The assertion of this form of knowledge has been found to have been based in a professional identity embraced by army medical practitioners during the Wars, which has been termed the 'military medical officer identity'. It has been shown that that identity was based on two concurrent processes: the evolution of medical theory based on overseas service and the need to assert competence in the face of professional hostility.

The first of these processes bears the most similarity to factors that have been shown to have been influential in the development of medical theories among practitioners who served in the East India Company and in the far reaches of the British Empire. The disease environments encountered by military medical officers on the Continent, in Egypt and in the West Indies challenged what they had learned at university and in classic medical texts, and their observations were incorporated into new theories of disease particularly in relation to dysentery, fevers and contagion. Some practitioners started to characterize the diseases suffered by the troops, as not sourced in individual constitutions or the environments in which they were operating, but in the behaviour and organization of the troops themselves. The need to cultivate military patrons both for career progression and to ensure that hygienic measures were enforced also prompted practitioners to incorporate values and concepts into their explanations of disease, and in particular their regimes of treatment, that embraced military values and organizational structures. Combined with the exigencies of practice in the difficult circumstances of a military campaign and the consequent limitations on what measures were practicable, these factors produced a medicine that was distinct. Although it bore a close relationship to 'tropical medicine' in its emphasis on climate, the importance of observation and experience, and strong shifts away from humoral explanations of disease – it was significantly militarized in both theory and application, and can be seen as a distinct branch of medicine, embracing the concepts of 'military disease' and a 'military specialty'. Within the military framework advocates of this military medicine; James McGrigor and allies of his, such as Francis Knight, endeavoured to establish best practice and to standardize the therapeutic approach to many diseases. Through such processes

McGrigor was significantly influential in the dissemination of the idea of military medicine throughout the force.

The second process reinforced the first and without it adherence to the idea that the practice of military medicine was specialized may not have been held to as strongly. Throughout the Wars, the officers of the AMD faced deprecation of their abilities, first from the pre-1810 AMB and later from physicians wedded to older forms of knowledge, the Portuguese medical administration and from civilian practitioners after the Wars. The effective barrier the pre-1810 Board placed in the path of promotion for military surgeons, and the increasingly apparent squeezing of the medical marketplace that would take place after the conclusion of the Wars, made it essential that military medical practitioners assert their claims to authority, expertise and marketplace share. This forced them to consider what made them special and what distinguished them from their competitors. It had the further effect of embedding many military practitioners more deeply within military structures and patronage networks as they sought alternative routes to promotion.

The assertions of their claims to authority were often articulated in published works, but I have argued that, more influentially, their approach was disseminated through assimilation into the British medical marketplace after the Wars and that their claims were often promoted to politicians and in Parliament. Considerations of parliamentary involvement in British medicine at this period have previously been confined to a few studies of the Walcheren inquiry and the 'Fifth Report', and to developments in sanitary medicine and medical police in the years after 1830. The preceding chapters have demonstrated that the parliamentary forum was utilized frequently by military medical officers, and that Parliament exhibited a strong interest in not only the administration of military medicine, but also in the theoretical basis underpinning various medical approaches. This compliments studies that have shown that many military practitioners began to use arguments designed to appeal to a government at War, particularly arguments based in manpower economy. The final chapter demonstrated that modes of medical rhetoric such as statistics, manpower economy arguments and the rational basis of observation-based medicine were aired repeatedly in Parliament over the course of the Wars, and it has been hypothesized that these forms of argument may have been seen to have been more persuasive to non-medically trained decision makers and that for that reason they were pursued by military medical officers. It has also been shown that by removing medical debates to this forum, medical practitioners ceded some of their authority to non-medical experts. However, it is in this forum that the principal claims for the influence of military medical practitioners in the promotion of empirical medicine have been advanced in this book.

By the end of the Wars, a large group of medical practitioners had emerged comprising men who considered themselves to be military medical officers. As a professional body they had militarized themselves and their medicine, and considered themselves a distinct professional body from their civilian counterparts. Throughout the Wars they had engaged in debates with civilian practitioners about many issues which all, ultimately, revolved around the central question of what type of knowledge should be considered most probative in medical debates. They deliberately attacked and sought to undermine the existing sites of medical authority. The empirical and observational model advocated by military medical officers underpinned their claims to authority and expertise and, after the Wars, for marketplace space over civilian practitioners. They disseminated this approach through their post-war practice and publications. They pursued their claims not only intra-professionally, but also in appeals to the public and in the parliamentary forum. By doing so they brought the issue outside the medical sphere and ceded some authority in the direction of British medicine to non-medical experts who are likely to have been more receptive to evidence based on empirical and observational models. Through all these means, the medical practitioners who served in the British army during the Wars had a significant impact on British medicine and its development over the next half-century.

NOTES

The following abbreviations have been used throughout the notes:

Add MS	Additional Manuscript (BL)
AMD	Army Medical Department
BL	British Library, London
CCR	Commons Committee Reports
ODNB	*Oxford Dictionary of National Biography*
EMSJ	*Edinburgh Medical and Surgical Journal*
GSC	Glasgow University Library Special Collections
HCSP	*House of Commons Sessional Papers*
RAMC	Royal Army Medical Corp series (WL)
TNA	The National Archives, London (formerly the Public Record Office)
Wars	The French Revolutionary and Napoleonic Wars
WL	Wellcome Library, London
WO	War Office Papers (TNA)

Introduction

1. M. Ackroyd, L. Brockliss, M. Moss, K. Retford and J. Stevenson, *Advancing with the Army, Medicine, the Professions, and Social Mobility in the British Isles, 1790–1850* (Oxford: Oxford University Press, 2006), pp. 44–5.
2. E. H. Ackerknecht, *Medicine at the Paris Hospital, 1794–1848* (Baltimore, MD: Johns Hopkins Press, 1967); and M. Foucault, *The Birth of the Clinic: An Archaeology of Medical Perception*, trans. A. M. Sheridan Smith (London: Tavistock, 1973).
3. D. Vess, *Medical Revolution in France, 1789–1796* (Gainsville, FL: University Presses of Florida, 1975); L. Brockliss and C. Jones, *The Medical World of Early Modern France* (Oxford: Clarendon Press, 1997), pp. 692–700.

4. M. Harrison, 'Disease and Medicine in the Armies of British India, 1750–1830: The Treatment of Fevers and the Emergence of Tropical Therapeutics', in G. L. Hudson (ed.), *British Military and Naval Medicine, 1600–1830* (Amsterdam and New York: Rodopi, 2007), pp. 87–119; K. F. Kiple, 'Race, War and Tropical Medicine in the Eighteenth-Century Caribbean', in D. Arnold (ed.), *Warm Climates and Western Medicine* (Amsterdam and Atlanta: Rodopi, 1996), pp. 65–79.

5. See for example: C. Hamlin, *Public Health and Social Justice in the Age of Chadwick, Britain, 1800–1854* (Cambridge: Cambridge University Press, 1998), pp. 53–8; C. Lawrence, *Medicine and the Making of Modern Britain 1700–1920* (London: Routledge, 1994).

6. J. V. Pickstone, 'Dearth, Dirt and Fever Epidemics: Rewriting the History of British "Public Health", 1780 1850', in T. Ranger and P. Slack (eds), *Epidemics and Ideas, Essays on the Historical Perception of Pestilence* (Cambridge: Cambridge University Press, 1992), pp. 125–48, on p. 141.

7. G. L. Hudson, 'Introduction, British Military and Naval Medicine, 1600–1830', in G. L. Hudson (ed.), *British Military and Naval Medicine*, pp. 7–22, on pp. 7–13.

8. M. Harrison, *Disease and the Modern World, 1500 to the Present Day* (Cambridge: Polity, 2004), p. 57; Brockliss and Jones, *The Medical World of Early Modern France*, pp. 689–700; D. P. Geggus, *Slavery, War and Revolution: The British Occupation of Saint Domingue 1793–1798* (Oxford and New York: Oxford University Press, 1982), pp. 347–72.

9. W. F. Bynum, 'Cullen and the Study of Fevers in Britain, 1760–1820', in W. F. Bynum and V. Nutton (eds), *Theories of Fever from Antiquity to the Enlightenment* (London: Wellcome Institute for the History of Medicine, 1981), pp. 135–47; P. Mathias, 'Swords into Ploughshares: The Armed Forces, Medicine and Public Health in the Late Eighteenth Century', in J. Winter (ed.), *War and Economic Development: Essays in Memory of David Joslin* (Cambridge: Cambridge University Press, 1975), pp. 73–90.

10. H. J. Cook, 'Practical Medicine and the British Armed Forces after the "Glorious Revolution"', *Medical History*, 34 (1990), pp. 1–26, on p. 13.

11. Ibid., p. 14.

12. C. Lawrence, 'Disciplining Diseases: Scurvy, the Navy and Imperial Expansion, 1750–1825', in D. Miller and P. Reill (eds), *Visions of Empire* (Cambridge: Cambridge University Press, 1996), pp. 80–106.

13. For the history of naval medicine in this period see generally: C. Lloyd and J. Coulter, *Medicine and the Navy, 1200–1900, 1714–1815*, 3 vols (Edinburgh: Livingstone, 1961), vol. 3; L. Brockliss, J. Cardwell and M. Moss, *Nelson's Surgeon, William Beatty, Naval Medicine, and the Battle of Trafalgar* (Oxford: Oxford University Press, 2005), ch. 1.

14. N. Cantlie, *A History of the Army Medical Department*, 2 vols (Edinburgh and London: Churchill Livingstone, 1974), vol. 1; a very similar treatment is provided in M. H. Kaufman, *Surgeons at War – Medical Arrangements for the Treatment of the Sick and Wounded in the British Army during the Late Eighteenth and Nineteenth Centuries* (Westport, CT: Greenwood Press, 2001). R. L. Blanco, 'The Development of British Military Medicine, 1793–1814', *Military Affairs*, 38 (1974), pp. 4–10; R. L. Blanco, *Wellington's Surgeon General: Sir James Macgrigor* (Durham, NC: Duke University Press, 1974); M. R. Howard, *Wellington's Doctors, The British Army Medical Services in the Napoleonic Wars* (Staplehurst: Spellmount, 2002).

15. See for example: Howard, *Wellington's Doctors*, p. 189.

16. Probably the best treatment by a military historian is: M. Glover, *Wellington's Army in the Peninsula 1808–1814* (London and Vancouver: David & Charles, 1977), ch. 10.

17. U. Tröhler, *'To Improve the Evidence of Medicine': The 18th Century British Origins of a Critical Approach* (Edinburgh: Royal College of Physicians of Edinburgh, 2000); see also E. M. Charters, 'Disease, War, and the Imperial State: The Health of the British Armed Forces during the Seven Years War, 1756–63' (D.Phil dissertation, University of Oxford, 2006), ch. 5.

18. Ackroyd et al., *Advancing with the Army*.

19. Ibid., p. 102.

20. See G. Weisz, 'The Emergence of Specialization in the Nineteenth Century', *Bulletin of the History of Medicine*, 77 (2003), pp. 536–75; G. Rosen, *The Specialization of Medicine with Particular Reference to Ophthalmology* (New York: Froben Press, 1944).

21. S. C. Lawrence, *Charitable Knowledge: Hospital Pupils and Practitioners in Eighteenth-Century London* (Cambridge: Cambridge University Press, 1996); I. Loudon, *Medical Care and the General Practitioner, 1750–1850* (Oxford: Clarendon Press, 1986); see also M. E. Fissell, *Patients, Power, and the Poor in Eighteenth-Century Bristol* (Cambridge: Cambridge University Press, 1991).

22. L. Rosner, *Medical Education in the Age of Improvement: Edinburgh Students and Apprentices, 1760–1826* (Edinburgh: Edinburgh University Press, 1991); M. H. Kaufman, *The Regius Chair of Military Surgery in the University of Edinburgh, 1806–55* (Amsterdam: Rodopi, 2003); L. S. Jacyna, *Philosophic Whigs: Medicine, Science and Citizenship in Edinburgh, 1789–1848* (London: Routledge, 1994).

1 The Low Countries and the West Indies

1. J. W. Fortescue, *A History of the British Army*, 13 vols (London: Macmillan, 1910–30), vol. 4, preface.

2. D. P. Geggus, 'Yellow Fever in the 1790s: The British Army in Occupied Saint Domingue', *Medical History*, 23 (1979), pp. 38–58; Kiple, 'Race, War and Tropical Medicine', pp. 65–79; Cantlie, *A History*, pp. 229–56.

3. Harrison, 'Disease and Medicine in the Armies of British India', pp. 87–119; M. Harrison, 'From Medical Astrology to Medical Astronomy: Sol-Lunar and Planetary Theories of Disease in British Medicine, c. 1700–1850', *British Journal for the History of Science*, 33 (2000), pp. 25–48, on p. 33; Geggus, 'Yellow Fever', pp. 53–6.

4. Geggus, 'Yellow Fever', p. 57.

5. Like all campaigns of this period, they are discussed in Cantlie, *A History*, pp. 210–29, and Fortescue, *A History*, pp. 80–324.

6. Cantlie, *A History*, p. 227. Cantlie's conclusions are echoed almost verbatim in Kaufman, *Surgeons at War*, p. 52.

7. Fortescue, *A History*, pp. 299–300.

8. R. Jackson, *An Outline of the History and Cure of Fever, Endemic and Contagious; More Expressly the Contagious Fever of Jails, Ships, and Hospitals; The Concentrated Endemic, Vulgarly the Yellow Fever of the West Indies. To which is Added, an Explanation of the Principles of Military Discipline and Economy; With a Scheme of Medical Arrangement for Armies* (Edinburgh: Printed for Mundell & Son, 1798), pp. 20–7; 'Borland to the Deputy Secretary at War', 28 December 1805, TNA, WO 40/22.

9. In September the sick rate amongst the British troops was 31 per cent. Cantlie, *A History*, p. 221.

10. Hunter was born near Glasgow in 1728 and moved to London in 1748 to assist his brother William Hunter, a successful teacher of anatomy and accoucheur. Despite embarking on several courses of study, by 1760 Hunter still did not qualify as a member of the Company of Surgeons. He joined the army as a staff surgeon in October 1760. After the Seven Years War he returned to London where over the next thirty years he was appointed to 'increasingly responsible and respectable offices of authority: as surgeon-extraordinary to the king in 1776, surgeon-general of the army, and inspector of its hospitals in 1790, positions earned as much by political skills and patronage as by qualification'. He died in 1793. J. Gruber, 'Hunter, John (1728–1793)', *ODNB*, online at http://www.oxforddnb.com/view/article/14220 [accessed 14 March 2008].

11. The characters and army service of these men are discussed extensively in Chapter 2. For biographical details see, G. Bettany, 'Gunning, John (*d.* 1798)', rev. M. Bevan, in *ODNB*, online at http://www.oxforddnb.com/view/article/11747 [accessed 14 March 2008]; G. Bettany, 'Keate, Thomas (1745–1821)', rev. M. Bevan, in *ODNB*, online at http://www.oxforddnb.com/view/article/15222 [accessed 14 March 2008]; and N. Moore, 'Pepys, Sir Lucas, first baronet (1742–1830)', rev. K. Bagshaw, *ODNB*, online at http://www.oxforddnb.com/view/article/21904 [accessed 14 March 2008].

12. Cantlie, *A History*, p. 227; see also Howard, *Wellington's Doctors*, p. 94.

13. 'Hunter to Amherst', 29 February 1793, TNA, WO 7/97, p. 101.

14. 'Keate to Gunning', 2 November 1793, TNA, WO 7/99, p. 7.

15. 'Keate and Gunning to General O'Hara', 7 December 1793, TNA, WO 7/100, p. 3.

16. See also the Board's claim that, 'The Complaints of want of Medical Abilities on our Entrance to Office were universal', 'AMB to Windham', undated, following a letter dated 29 June 1795, TNA, WO 7/102, p. 9.

17. R. Hamilton, *The Duties of a Regimental Surgeon Considered with Observations on his General Qualifications; And Hints Relative to a More Respectable Practice, and Better Regulation of that Department*, 2nd edn (London: printed by George Woodfall, for T. N. Longman; J. Johnson; and P. Foster, Ipswich, 1794), p. ix.

18. Ibid., pp. 79–80.

19. Ibid., p. 81.

20. 'Keate to Gunning', 2 November 1793, TNA, WO 7/99, p. 7; 'AMB to Amherst', 31 March, 1794, TNA, WO 7/101, pp. 39–40.

21. Hamilton, *The Duties of a Regimental Surgeon*, p. 289.

22. See for example: 'Keate to Bowles', 25 November 1793, TNA, WO 7/99, p. 54; 'Keate to Shapter', 6 December 1793, TNA, WO 7/100, p. 10; 'Keate to Grieves', undated, following a letter dated 9 June 1794, TNA, WO 7/101, p. 155; 'Emerson to Coombs', 11 June 1796, TNA, WO 7/104, p. 30.

23. 'Keate to St Leger', 3 December 1793, TNA, WO 7/99, p. 68.

24. 'AMB to Abercrombie', 28 March 1796, TNA, WO 7/103, p. 90.

25. N. Sinnott, *Observations, Tending to Shew the Mismanagement of the Medical Department in the Army; With a View to Trace the Evils to their Source: And to Point out to Government the Necessity of Attending More to the Health of the Soldier in Time of War. To which is Annexed, a Representation of the System Adopted in the Hanoverian Service* (London: For J. Murray & S. Highley, 1796), pp. 9–15.

26. 'Borland to the Deputy Secretary at War', 28 December 1805, TNA, WO 40/22.

27. J. Fergusson (ed.), *William Fergusson, Notes and Recollections of a Professional Life* (London: Longman, Brown, Green & Longmans, 1846), p. 58.

28. D. Monro, *Observations on the Means of Preserving the Health of Soldiers*, 2nd edn, 2 vols (London: John Murray, 1780); J. Pringle, *Observations on the Diseases of the Army*, 6th edn (London: Printed for A. Millar & T. Cadell, D. Wilson, T. Durham and T. Payne, 1768).

29. 'Younge to duke of York', 8 May 1793, TNA, WO 4/291, p. 55.

30. Kennedy was at this time physician to St Bartholomew's Hospital, and had previously served as a physician to the forces during the American War of Independence. Cantlie, *A History*, p. 213.

31. 'Hunter to Amherst', 28 June 1793, TNA, WO 7/98, p. 25.

32. 'Hunter to Amherst', 29 August 1793, TNA, WO 7/98, p. 31.

33. Home (1756–1832) was the son of an army surgeon. Educated as a King's scholar at Westminster School, he gained a scholarship to Trinity College, Cambridge, in 1773, but decided instead to become a surgical pupil of his brother-in-law John Hunter. He qualified through the Company of Surgeons in 1778 and was appointed assistant surgeon in the naval hospital at Plymouth. In 1779 he served as a staff surgeon with the army in Jamaica, returned to England on half pay in 1784 and rejoined Hunter at St George's Hospital as assistant in teaching, research and clinical practice. He was elected FRS on 15 February 1787 and in the same year became assistant surgeon at St George's Hospital. In 1790–1 Home read lectures for Hunter and in the following year he succeeded Hunter as lecturer in anatomy. He went on to have a successful and illustrious career, despite questions over whether he represented Hunter's findings as his own after Hunter's death. N. Coley, 'Home, Sir Everard, first baronet (1756–1832)', *ODNB*, online at http://www.oxforddnb.com/view/article/13639 [accessed 16 March 2008].

34. 'Report of Mr Home', 30 September 1793, TNA, WO 4/291, p. 121.

35. Ibid., p. 120

36. Ibid., p. 122.

37. 'Keate to St Leger', undated, following a letter dated 5 November 1793, TNA, WO 7/99, p. 34.

38. 'Keate to St Leger', 19 November 1793, TNA, WO 7/99, p. 42.

39. 'Gunning and Keate to Amherst', 28 November 1793, TNA, WO 7/99, p. 57.

40. Ibid.

41. 'Gunning and Keate to Amherst', 1 January 1794, TNA, WO 7/100, p. 37.

42. 'Amherst to Gunning and Keate', 2 January 1794, TNA, WO 7/100, p. 50.

43. 'Gunning to Kennedy', 6 January 1794, TNA, WO 7/100, pp. 46–7.

44. 'AMB to John Macnamara Hayes', 8 January 1794, TNA, WO 7/100, p. 49.

45. 'Keate to St Leger', 13 January 1794, TNA, WO 7/100, p. 54.

46. Ibid., p. 55.

47. 'Dickson to his sister', 15 July 1794, in A. Cormack, *James Dickson, M. A. 1769–1795 Army Surgeon* (Aberdeenshire, 1968), WL, RAMC 715/5, p. 68.

48. 'Keate to West', 2 June 1794, TNA, WO 7/101, p. 149.

49. 'AMB to Amherst', 11 February 1794, TNA, WO 7/101, p. 78; 'AMB to Kennedy', 13 May 1794, TNA, 7/101, p.117.

50. 'AMB to Amherst', 19 February 1794, TNA, WO 7/100, pp. 84–5.

51. 'Amherst to AMB', 19 February 1794, TNA, WO 7/100, p. 85.

52. Hunter had studied at Edinburgh and he graduated MD in 1775. He was admitted a licentiate of the Royal College of Physicians in London on 22 March 1777, after which he was appointed physician to the army, through the influence of Sir George Baker and William Heberden. From 1781 to 1783 he was superintendent of the military hospitals

in Jamaica. After returning to England he settled in practice as a physician in London. Hunter is best known for his *Observations on the Diseases of the Army in Jamaica*, which appeared in 1788. He was admitted a fellow of the Royal College of Physicians *speciali gratia* in 1793. C. Creighton, 'Hunter, John (1754–1809)', rev. L. Wilkinson, *ODNB*, online at http://www.oxforddnb.com/view/article/14221 [accessed 16 March 2008].

53. 'Keate to Secretary at War', 22 February 1794, TNA, WO 7/101, p. 4; 'Amherst to Pepys', 24 February 1794, TNA, WO 7/101, p. 7.

54. 'Keate to Hunter', 13 March 1794, TNA, WO 7/101, p. 24.

55. 'Keate's Report on the Chatham Hospitals', undated, following a letter 25 March 1794, TNA, WO 7/101, p. 30.

56. 'Keate to Amherst', 29 March 1794, TNA, WO 7/101, p. 47.

57. Ibid.

58. 'Lennox to Secretary at War', 4 February 1794, TNA, WO 1/896, pp. 11–15.

59. Jerome Fitzpatrick was a noted Irish physician and campaigner for prison reform. He was sent to Flanders in the winter of 1794 to assist with the medical crisis there, and was very critical of Kennedy's medical arrangements. See J. Kelly, 'Fitzpatrick, Sir Jeremiah (*c.* 1740–1810)', in *ODNB*, online at http://www.oxforddnb.com/view/article/61603 [accessed 16 March 2008]; and R. L. Blanco, 'The Soldier's Friend – Sir Jeremiah Fitzpatrick, Inspector of Health for Land Forces', *Medical History*, 20 (1976), pp. 402–21; Cantlie, *A History*, pp. 223–7; O. MacDonagh, *The Inspector General: Sir Jeremiah Fitzpatrick and the Politics of Social Reform, 1783–1802* (London: Croom Helm, 1981).

60. 'Fitzpatrick to Lennox', 23 January 1794, TNA, WO 1/896, pp. 19–23; 'Fitzpatrick to Lennox', undated, TNA, WO 1/896, pp. 27–9; 'Fitzpatrick to Lennox', undated, TNA, WO 1/896, pp. 31–8.

61. Throughout TNA, WO 1/896 to p. 78.

62. 'AMB to Secretary at War', 3 May 1794, TNA, WO 1/896, pp. 78–82.

63. 'Lennox to Secretary at War', 7 December 1794, TNA, WO 1/896, p. 123.

64. Cantlie, *A History*, pp. 219–20.

65. 'Craig to Secretary at War', private, 19 July 1794, TNA, WO 1/169, p. 927; see also 'Craig to Amherst', 12 August 1794, TNA, WO 1/170, p. 177.

66. 'Craig to [unknown – Commander in Chief?]', 27 November 1794, TNA, WO 1/171, p. 334.

67. 'Harcourt to duke of York', 15 December 1794, TNA, WO 1/171, p. 484.

68. 'Harcourt to duke of York', 18 December 1794, TNA, WO, 1/171, pp. 553–62.

69. 'Harcourt to duke of York', 21 January 1795, TNA, WO 1/172, p. 168.

70. 'Harcourt to duke of York', 11 February 1795, TNA, WO 1/172, pp. 246–7.

71. R. Jackson, *A System of Arrangement and Discipline, for the Medical Department of Armies* (London: John Murray, 1805), p. xiii.

72. R. Jackson, *A Treatise on the Fevers of Jamaica, with some Observations on the Intermitting Fever of America, and an Appendix Containing some Hints on the Means of Preserving the Health of Soldiers in Hot Climates* (London: John Murray, 1791).

73. These aspects of Jackson's philosophy are set out throughout his works, particularly Jackson, *A System* and Jackson, *A Treatise on the Fevers of Jamaica*. For discussion see N. Saakwa-Mante, 'Jackson, Robert (*bap.* 1750, *d.* 1827)', *ODNB*, online at http://www.oxforddnb.com/view/article/14547 [accessed 16 March 2008].

74. In 1799, Calvert became adjutant general to the forces and is noted for his contribution to the administration and discipline of the army, including the organization of the medical department and army hospitals. H. Chichester, 'Calvert, Sir Harry, first baronet (*bap.*

1763, *d.* 1826)', rev. J. Sweetman, *ODNB*, online at http://www.oxforddnb.com/view/article/4422 [accessed 16 March 2008].

75. 'Calvert to Dalrymple', 28 September 1794, in H. Verney (ed.), *The Journals and Correspondence of General Sir Harry Calvert, Bart ... Comprising the Campaigns in Flanders and Holland in 1793–4* (London: Hurst & Blackett, 1853), p. 337.

76. 'Calvert to Dalrymple', 24 October 1794, in Verney, *The Journals*, p. 367.

77. 'AMB to Balfour', undated, following a letter 17 March 1794, TNA, WO 7/101, p. 39.

78. Cantlie, *A History*, p. 226; Sinnott, *Observations*, p. 17.

79. 'AMB to Windham', undated, following a letter 29 June 1795, TNA, WO 7/102, p. 10.

80. 'Harcourt to duke of York', 18 April 1795, TNA, WO 1/172, p. 43.

81. 'AMB to Windham', undated, following letter 29 June 1795, TNA, WO 7/102, pp. 10–12.

82. See, for example, Sinnott, *Observations*, p. 17.

83. 'AMB to Windham', 27 April 1795, regarding General Stewart's expedition to Corsica, TNA, WO 7/102, pp. 3–4; 'AMB to Windham', regarding Sir Charles Grey in the West Indies, TNA, WO 7/102, pp. 4–5; 'AMB to Windham', 8 July 1795, regarding Sir John Vaughn's command in the West Indies, TNA, WO 7/102, p. 12; 'AMB to Brownrigg', 30 January 1796, regarding colonels in the East Indies, TNA, WO 7/102, p. 37.

84. 'AMB to Windham', 3 June 1797, TNA, WO 7/105, p. 100.

85. 'AMB to Lewis', 6 May 1797, TNA, WO 7/105, p. 85.

86. 'AMB to Windham', 23 March 1795, TNA, WO 7/102, p. 4.

87. 'AMB to Lewis', 13 February 1797, TNA, WO 7/105, p. 13.

88. Harrison, *Disease and the Modern World*, p. 57; Geggus, *Slavery, War and Revolution*, pp. 347–72.

89. Kiple, 'Race, War and Tropical Medicine', pp. 66–7; Bynum, 'Cullen and the Study of Fevers in Britain', p. 142.

90. Jackson, *An Outline of the History and Cure of Fever*; 'Borland to the Deputy Secretary at War', 28 December 1805, TNA, WO 40/22; See also, 'Dissertatio meduca ubauguralis de typhi remediis, Auctore Baldwin Wake' *EMSJ*, 4 (1808), pp. 117–20.

91. Jackson, *An Outline of the History and Cure of Fever*, p. 20.

92. Monro, *Observations*; Pringle, *Observations*; J. Lind, *An Essay on Diseases Incidental to Europeans in Hot Climates with the Method of Preventing Their Fatal Consequences* (London: T. Becket & P. A. de Hondt, 1768); see also Harrison, 'Disease and Medicine in the Armies of British India', pp. 92–93l.

93. Lawrence, 'Disciplining Diseases'.

94. The similarities between Jackson's identification of army culture as a source of disease and a shift from atmospheric to sanitary/cultural explanations of disease in India at the beginning of the nineteenth century should also be noted, see M. Harrison, *Climates and Constitutions: Health, Race, Environment and British Imperialism in India 1600–1850* (New Delhi: Oxford University Press, 1999), ch. 4.

95. M. McGrigor (ed.), *Sir James McGrigor. The Scalpel and the Sword. The Autobiography of the Father of Army Medicine* (Dalkeith: Scottish Cultural Press, 2000), p. 43.

96. W. Fergusson, 'A Letter to the Managers of the Royal Infirmary Edinburgh' (Edinburgh, 1818), WL, RAMC 474/61, pp. 14–16.

97. Ibid.

98. On the medical arrangements for the campaigns generally see, Cantlie, *A History*, pp. 229–45. For a discussion of the reasons behind the virulence of yellow fever during these years, and an estimate of the losses suffered see Geggus, 'Yellow Fever'.

99. M. Harrison, *Medicine in an Age of Commerce and Empire Britain and its Tropical Colonies 1660–1830* (Oxford: Oxford University Press, 2010).
100. Fergusson, *William Fergusson, Notes and Recollections*, p. 153.
101. Geggus, 'Yellow Fever', p. 55.
102. Jackson, *An Outline of the History and Cure of Fever*.
103. H. McLean, *An Enquiry into the Nature, and Causes of the Great Mortality Among the Troops at St. Domingo: With Practical Remarks on the Fever of that Island* (London: Printed for T. Cadell, 1797).
104. Ibid., p. xvi.
105. Ibid., p. 226
106. Ibid., pp. 239–40; see also p. 244.
107. W. Lempriere, *Practical Observations on the Diseases of the Army in Jamaica, As they Occurred Between the Years 1792 and 1797*, 2 vols (London: T. N. Longman & O. Rees, 1799).

2 Walcheren and the Army Medical Board

1. For details of the Board's arrangement and division of responsibilities, see 'Fifth Report of the Commissioners of Military Enquiry', *HCSP*, 5 (1808), pp. 4–7; and A. Peterkin, W. Johnston and R. Drew, *Commissioned Officers in the Medical Services of the British Army, 1660–1960* (London: Wellcome Historical Medical Library, 1968), pp. xlviii–l.
2. C. Hibbert (ed.), *The Recollections of Rifleman Harris as told to Henry Curling* (London: Century, 1985), p. 115.
3. *Cobbett's Parliamentary Debates*, 16, p. 406: 30 March 1810, per Mr Bathurst.
4. Details of the Walcheren Campaign are recorded in papers of the House of Commons inquiry into the expedition, 'Papers Presented to the House, by His Majesty's Command Relating to the Expedition To The Scheldt', *HCSP*, 6–8 (1810); and 'Papers Relating to the Army Medical Board', *HCSP*, 14 (1810).
5. Details of the expedition can be found throughout *HCSP*, 6 (1810).
6. *HCSP*, 6 (1810), p. 29.
7. *HCSP*, 6 (1810), p. 92.
8. *HCSP*, 6 (1810), pp. 92, 125.
9. *HCSP*, 8 (1810), pp. 16–20 (evidence of Sir Lucas Pepys); pp. 21–33 (Thomas Keate, Esq.); pp. 33–5 (Francis Knight).
10. *Cobbett's Parliamentary Debates*, 16, p. 422: 30 March 1810.
11. See for consideration of various aspects of the AMD and its dealings related to the Walcheren campaign: Cantlie, *A History*, pp. 183–209, 395–405; Blanco, 'The Development of British Military Medicine', pp. 4–10; R. Feibel, 'What Happened at Walcheren: The Primary Medical Sources', *Bulletin of the History of Medicine*, 42 (1968), pp. 62–79, for a detailed investigation of the nature of the disease; G. Kempthorne, 'The Walcheren Expedition and the Reform of the Medical Board, 1809', *Journal of the Royal Army Medical Corps*, 62 (1934), pp. 133–8.
12. A. Chaplin, *Medicine in England during the Reign of George the Third* (London: published by the author, 1919), p. 86; K. Crowe, 'The Walcheren Expedition and the New Army Medical Board: A Reconsideration', *English Historical Review*, 88 (1973), pp. 770–85. See also, 'Fifth Report', p. 82.
13. *HCSP*, 14 (1810), pp. 159–80, 195, 203–15.
14. Sinnott, *Observations*.

15. J. Bell, *Memorial Concerning the Present State of Military and Naval Surgery Addressed Several Years Ago to the Right Honorable Earl Spencer, First Lord of the Admiralty; And Now Submitted to the Public* (Edinburgh: Longman & Rees, 1800).

16. Sir Lucas Pepys (1742–1830) was educated at Eton College and at Christ Church, Oxford, where he graduated his BA on 9 May 1764. He then studied medicine at Edinburgh in 1765, and afterwards graduated at Oxford, MA on 13 May 1767, MB on 30 April 1770, and MD on 14 June 1774. Pepys was elected a fellow of the Royal College of Physicians on 30 September 1775, and was president from 1804 to 1810. In 1777, he was appointed physician-extraordinary to the King, and in 1792 physician-in-ordinary. He was created a baronet on 22 January 1784. Moore, 'Pepys, Sir Lucas, first baronet (1742–1830)', rev. K. Bagshaw, *ODNB*. Thomas Keate (1745–1821) was a pupil at St George's Hospital, London, and from 1787 was assistant to John Gunning, surgeon to the hospital. He became regimental surgeon of the foot guards in 1778 and served as inspector of regimental infirmaries until 1798. He succeeded Gunning in 1798 as surgeon-general to the army, and was elected a fellow of the Royal Society in 1799. He was surgeon to the Prince of Wales, afterwards George IV, and to Chelsea Hospital. Bettany, 'Keate, Thomas (1745–1821)', rev. M. Bevan, *ODNB*.

17. See *HCSP*, 14 (1810), p. 180: Physician general to the secretary at war, 28 January 1810: 'The regular Physicians from those Universities were gradually getting into charge of the Army. This I have been bringing about for the last sixteen years'. See also 'Fifth Report', appendix 5, p. 99: 'Examination of Sir Lucas Pepys' in which he also acknowledged that he had no personal experience of military medicine.

18. For an account of Jackson's practices on the Isle of Wight see *Proceedings and Report of a Special Medical Board Appointed by His Royal Highness the Commander in Chief, and the Secretary at War to Examine the State of the Hospital at the Military Depot in the Isle of Wight, &c. &c. &c.* (London: L. B. Seeley, 1808).

19. Ibid., p. 13.

20. Ibid., p. 32.

21. Ibid., p. 32.

22. Ibid., p. 60.

23. Ibid., p. 65.

24. R. Jackson, *Remarks on the Constitution of the Medical Department of the British Army: With a Detail of Hospital Management, and an Appendix, Attempting to Explain the Action of Causes in Producing Fever, and the Operation of Remedies in Effecting Cure* (London: T. Cadell & W. Davies, 1803); R. Jackson, *A Systematic View of the Formation, Discipline, and Economy of Armies* (London: John Stockdale, 1804); Jackson, *A System of Arrangement and Discipline*.

25. Jackson, *A System of Arrangement and Discipline*, pp. xvii, 55, 84–91, 450–4.

26. Ibid., p. xvii; For Knight's service see Peterkin et al., *Commissioned Officers*, p. 55.

27. For evidence of the growing division between Pepys/Keate and Knight/Jackson/Borland see *HCSP*, 14 (1810), pp. 186–94: surgeon general to the secretary at war, 4 August 1809.

28. 'Fifth Report', p. 3.

29. See Jackson, *A Treatise on the Fevers of Jamaica*, pp. 420–4; Jackson, *A System of Arrangement and Discipline*, pp. 12, 50153–163, 459; R. Jackson, *A Letter to the Commissioners of Military Enquiry; Explaining the True Constitution of a Medical Staff, the Best Form of Economy for Hospitals &c. With a Refutation of Errors and Misrepresentations Contained*

in a letter by Dr Bancroft Army Physician, dated 28 April 1808 (London: the author, 1808), pp. 34–55; Fergusson, *William Fergusson, Notes and Recollections*, pp. 58–61.

30. See T. Keate, *Observations on the Fifth Report of the Commissioners of Military Enquiry and More Particularly on Those Parts of it which Relate to the Surgeon General* (London: J. Hatchard, 1808), pp. 45–54, 59.

31. Sinnott, *Observations*, pp. 15–28.

32. E. Bancroft, *A Letter to the Commissioners of Military Enquiry: Containing Animadversions on Some Parts of Their Fifth Report; And an Examination of the Principles on which the Medical Department of the Armies Ought to be Formed* (London: T. Cadell & W. Davies, 1808), pp. 1–20; *HCSP*, 14 (1810), p. 180: 'Letter from the Physician General to the Secretary at War', 28 January, 1810.

33. McGrigor, *Sir James McGrigor. The Scalpel and the Sword*, pp. 125–6.

34. 'Fifth Report', p. 5.

35. See L. Rosner, *The Most Beautiful Man in Existence: The Scandalous Life of Alexander Lesassier* (Philadelphia: University of Pennsylvania Press, 1999), pp. 11–12, 32, 195, for an excellent portrait of the motivations of many young men who chose to enter medicine and the AMD during this period; see also Chapter 5.

36. 'Fifth Report', p. 22.

37. Ibid., p. 81.

38. Ibid., p.16.

39. Ibid., pp. 24–8.

40. Ibid., p. 23.

41. Ibid., p. 77.

42. Keate, *Observations on the Fifth Report*.

43. Ibid., p. 11.

44. Ibid., pp. 15–18.

45. Ibid., pp. 41–5; see also S. Shapin, *A Social History of Truth: Civility and Science in Seventeenth-Century England* (Chicago, IL: University of Chicago Press, 1994), for an indication of the seriousness of such an accusation during the early nineteenth century.

46. Keate, *Observations*, p. 30.

47. Ibid., p. 29.

48. Ibid.

49. Ibid., p. 57.

50. Ibid., appendix 8, p. B2.

51. J. Borland, 'Copy of a Letter from Dr. Borland, to the Inspector Generals of Army Hospitals; dated 20th June 1808', in *Papers relating to the Army Medical Board* (Ordered by the House of Commons to be printed 4 May 1810: London, 1810).

52. Ibid., p. 121.

53. Ibid., p. 126.

54. R. Jackson, *A Letter to Mr Keate, Surgeon General to the Forces* (London: John Murray, 1808).

55. Jackson, *A Letter to the Commissioners of Military Enquiry*.

56. Ibid., p. 15.

57. However, see his views on yellow fever as set out in Harrison, *British Medicine in an Age of Commerce*.

58. Edward Nathaniel Bancroft (1772–1842), graduated BM from St John's College, Cambridge, in 1794. In 1795, he was appointed a physician to the forces. Bancroft served in the Windward Islands, in Portugal, in the Mediterranean, and in Egypt. On his return to England he obtained an MD from Cambridge, in 1804. He joined the Royal College of

Physicians in 1805, became a fellow in 1806. C. Creighton, 'Bancroft, Edward Nathaniel (1772–1842)', rev. J. Reznick, *ODNB*, online at http://www.oxforddnb.com/view/article/1268 [accessed 23 March 2008].

59. Bancroft, *A Letter to the Commissioners*, p. 2.
60. Ibid., p. 8.
61. Ibid., p. 12.
62. Ibid., pp. 17–19.
63. Ibid., p. 61.
64. Ibid., p. 63. Yates had begun service with the Medical Department of the East India Company as an assistant surgeon in 1795 and became surgeon in course of seniority. He served in the general hospital at Calcutta, was detached to Ceylon, and was eventually appointed garrison surgeon at Point de Galle, where he served seven years. During his service in Calcutta he worked closely with Charles Maclean (see Chapter 6). See 'Fifth Report', p. 190.
65. Bancroft, *A Letter to the Commissioners*, pp. 80–2.
66. Ibid., p. 82.
67. Ibid., p. 101.
68. J. McGrigor, *A Letter to the Commissioners of Military Enquiry, In reply to Some Animadversions of Dr E. Nathaniel Bancroft on their Fifth Report* (London: John Murray, 1808).
69. Ibid., p. 2.
70. Shapin, *A Social History of Truth*.
71. McGrigor, *A Letter to the Commissioners of Military Enquiry*, p. 31.
72. Ibid., p. 5.
73. Ibid., p. 51.
74. Jackson, *A Letter to the Commissioners of Military Enquiry*.
75. E. Bancroft, *An Exposure and Refutation of Various Misrepresentations Published by Dr McGrigor and Dr Jackson, in their Separate Letters to the Commissioners of Military Enquiry; Interspersed with Facts and Observations Concerning Military Hospitals and Medical Arrangements for Armies* (London: T. Cadell & W. Davies, 1808).
76. Anon., 'Of the Practice of Medicine in Great Britain, as Conducted by Physicians, Surgeons, Apothecaries, &c. &c.', *Medical Observer*, 1 (1806), p. 195.
77. 'Arataeus' Review of publications respecting the medical department of the army', *Medical Observer*, 3 (1808), p. 214. Dr Charles Maclean claims to have been the author of this letter in his, *An Analytical View of the Medical Department of the British Army* (London: J. J. Stockdale, 1810), p. iv.
78. W. Nisbet., 'On the 5th Report of the Commissioners of Military Enquiry, on the Medical Department of the Army', *London Medical and Surgical Spectator*, 1 (1808), pp. 122–31, on p.127.
79. See in this regard Rosner, *The Most Beautiful Man*, in which the medical practitioner Alexander Lesassier exhibits a clear preference for work in general hospitals for the reason, *inter alia*, that in them, he was more likely to be noticed by powerful men and gain advancement.
80. 'Secretary at War, to the Physician General', 12th May 1808, *HCSP*, 14 (1810), p. 203.
81. 'Surgeon General to the Secretary at War', 28 July 1808, *HCSP*, 14 (1810), p. 203.
82. 'Physician General and the Surgeon General to the Secretary at War', 3 January 1809, *HCSP*, 14 (1810), pp. 218–20.
83. 'Commander in Chief to the Secretary at War', 26 June 1809, *HCSP*, 14 (1810), pp. 200–1.

84. 'Francis Knight to F. Moore', 1 August, 1809, *HCSP*, 6 (1810), p. 146.
85. Cantlie states that the constitution of the board was at the initiative of Francis Knight, *A History*, p. 308.
86. 'Commander in Chief to the Secretary at War', 26 June 26 1809, *HCSP*, 14 (1810), pp. 200–1.
87. 'Inspector General of Army Hospitals, to the Secretary at War', 18 July 1809, *HCSP*, 14 (1810), pp. 153–4; 'Francis Knight to F. Moore', 1 August, 1809, see also *HCSP*, 6 (18100, p. 146; and 'Francis Knight to F. Moore', 21 July 1809, *HCSP*, 6 (1810), p. 143.
88. *HCSP*, 14 (1810), pp. 187–93.
89. 'Lt Col. Gordon, to Francis Moore, Esq.', 4 August 1809, *HCSP*, 7 (1810), p. 11; 'Deputy Secretary at War to the Principal Officers of the AMD', 5 August 1809, *HCSP*, 7 (1810), p. 286.
90. 'Francis Knight, Esq. to the Adjutant General', 6 August 1809, *HCSP*, 14 (1810), p. 199.
91. 'Inspector General of Army Hospitals, to the Deputy Secretary at War', 7 August 1809, *HCSP*, 14 (1810), pp. 199–200.
92. 'William Huskinsson, Esq. to the Secretary at War', 8 August 1809, *HCSP*, 14 (1810), p. 151; 'Deputy Secretary at War to Lieut. Colonel Gordon', 10 August 1809, *HCSP*, 14 (1810), p. 158.
93. 'Deputy Secretary at War to the Principal Officers of the AMD', 15 August 1809, *HCSP*, 7 (1810), p. 286.
94. 'Francis Moore, Esq. to Lieut Col. Gordon', 9 September, 1809, *HCSP*, 6 (1810), p. 169; 'Thomas Keate to Francis Moore', 11 September 1809, *HCSP*, 6 (1810), p. 174; 'Thomas Keate to Francis Moore', 11 September 1809, *HCSP*, 6 (1810), p. 175; 'Lucas Pepys to Francis Moore', 13 September 1809, *HCSP*, 6 (1810), p. 181.
95. 'Francis Moore to the AMD', 25 September 1809, *HCSP*, 7 (1810), p. 46.
96. 'Knight to Moore', 25 September 1809, *HCSP*, 7 (1810), p. 46.
97. 'Dundas to Coote', 26 September 1809, *HCSP*, 6 (1810), p. 198.
98. 'Pepys to Moore', 27 September, 1809, *HCSP*, 7 (1810), p. 47.
99. 'Moore to Pepys', 27 September 1809, *HCSP*, 7 (1810), p. 48.
100. 'Physician General to the Deputy Secretary at War', 27 September 1809, *HCSP*, 7 (1810), p. 54.
101. 'Moore to the AMD', 28 September 1809, *HCSP*, 7 (1810), p. 49.
102. 'Knight to Moore', 28 September, 1809, *HCSP*, 7 (1810), p. 48.
103. 'Blane to AMD', 2 October 1809, *HCSP*, 6 (1810), p. 91; 'Blane to AMD', 6 October 1809, *HCSP*, 6 (1810), pp. 228–9.
104. 'Moore to Col. Torrens', 13 October, 1809, *HCSP*, 6 (1810), p. 227.
105. 'Blane to Pepys', 9 October 1809, *HCSP*, 6 (1810), p. 241.
106. 'Keate to Moore', 6 October 1809, *HCSP*, 7 (1810), p. 324.
107. McGrigor, *Sir James McGrigor. The Scalpel and the Sword*, p. 158.
108. 'Commander in Chief to the Secretary at War', 30 December 1809, *HCSP*, 14 (1810), p. 160.
109. 'Pepys to Major General Calvert, Adjutant General of the Forces', 8 December 1809, *HCSP*, 7 (1810), pp. 275–6; 'Surgeon General to the Deputy Secretary at War', 14 December 1809, *HCSP*, 7 (1810), pp. 297–8.
110. 'Surgeon General to the Secretary at War', 8 January 1810, *HCSP*, 14 (1810), p. 166; 'Physician General to the Secretary at War', 7 January 1810, *HCSP*, 14 (1810), p. 168.
111. 'Physician General to the Secretary at War', 28 January 1810, *HCSP*, 14 (1810), p. 180.

112. See 'Examination of Sir Lucas Pepys', *HCSP*, 8 (1810), p. 17; 'Examination of Francis Knight, Esq.', *HCSP*, 8 (1810), p. 34; 'Examination of James McGrigor, M.D.', *HCSP*, 8 (1810), p. 260.

113. See 'Examination of Sir Lucas Pepys', *HCSP*, 8 (1810), pp. 16, 18; 'Examination of Thomas Keate, Esq.', HCSP, 8 (1810), p. 9.

114. *HCSP*, 8 (1810), pp. 253–9.

115. See for example, *Cobbett's Parliamentary Debates*, 15 (1810), p. 162: per Lord Porchester, 26 January 1810; p. 185: per Mr Fuller, 26 January 1810; p. 207: per Mr Canning, 26 January 1810. See also, *The Times Digital Archive, 1785–1985*, Thompson Gale Databases, 14 November 1809, p. 2; and *The Times Digital Archive*, 2 February 1810, p. 3.

3 Egypt, Ophthalmia and Plague

1. The expedition numbered 56,000 men in all: 36,000 being troops and the rest made up of Napoleon's personal guard, auxiliary staff and the Commission of the Arts and Sciences. For a military account of the French expedition see J. R. Cole, *Napoleon's Egypt: Invading the Middle East* (New York and Basingstoke: Palgrave MacMillan, 2007); for a general account see: D. Chandler, 'The Egyptian Campaign of 1801, Part 1', *History Today*, 12 (February 1962), pp. 16–123; and 'The Egyptian Campaign of 1801, Part 2', *History Today*, 12 (March 1962), pp. 177–86.

2. The best account of the British expedition is: R. Wilson, *History of the British Expedition to Egypt; To which is Subjoined, A Sketch of the Present State of that Country and its Means of Defence. Illustrated with Maps, and a Portrait of Sir Ralph Abercromby*, 2nd edn (London: C. Roworth, 1803); for a modern account of the British expedition see P. Macksey, *British Victory in Egypt, 1801: The End of Napoleon's Conquest* (London: Routledge, 1995).

3. B. Simms, 'Britain & Napoleon', *Historical Journal*, 41 (1998), pp. 885–94, on p. 892.

4. In his seminal work on the development of medical specialization, *The Specialization of Medicine with Particular Reference to Ophthalmology*, George Rosen argued that around the mid-nineteenth century ophthalmology, which had been largely ignored or derided prior to that time, emerged as 'one of the first medical specialties' (p. 50). Although he did not specifically identify the Egyptian ophthalmia as a catalyst for that development he argued that the emergence of specialist eye hospitals in the second decade of the nineteenth century must 'be considered of prime importance' (p. 32); in his, *The History of Ophthalmology Translated by Frederick C. Blodi, M. D.* (Bonn: Wayenborgh, 1985) Julius Hirschberg argued that until 1820 there was no complete textbook of 'ophthalmy' in English, and that around the turn of the century 'ophthalmy' was virtually ignored in England. Referring to the spread of ophthalmia through the British Army and civilian population following the expedition to Egypt, he stated that 'The main impetus to improve English Ophthalmy during the beginning of the nineteenth century was dire need', and that the symptoms of the disease 'must have presented a tremendous challenge to English surgeons'. He also stated that the specialist eye hospitals which were founded around this time were partially a response to that crisis (vol. 8a, p. 8). The issue was reconsidered by L. Davidson, '"Identities Ascertained": British Ophthalmology in the First Half of the Nineteenth Century', *Social History of Medicine*, 9 (1996), pp. 313–33. Davidson builds on the work of Rosen to demonstrate the cultural and moral resonances of Egyptian ophthalmia and the ways in which they were employed by surgeons to develop the authority of 'eye medicine' as a specialty.

5.   Cantlie, *A History*, pp. 264–81; G. Kempthorne, 'The Egyptian Campaign of 1801', *Journal of the Royal Army Medical Corps*, 55 (1930), pp. 217–30.

6.   Blanco, *Wellington's Surgeon General*, ch. 7; R.G. Richardson, *Larrey, Surgeon to Napoleon's Imperial Guard* (London: Quiller Press, 2000), chs 6–10.

7.   P. Alpinus, *La médicine des Egyptiens 1581–1584 traduite du latin, et anotée par R. de Fenol* (Cairo: Institut francais d'archaeologie orientale du Caire, 1980). Grounded in a Galenic view of disease, Alpinus also set out in detail the approach of the native Egyptians to the cure of their endemic diseases, including plague and an inflammation of the eyes. Much of Alpinus's analysis of the cause of disease in Egypt accorded significant influence to the climate, its extremes of heat and cold, the effects of the winds and the Nile's annual flood. He argued that the inflammation of the eyes was caused by the 'poussière nitreuse' in the air, and reported that to preserve themselves the local people washed their eyes many times a day with cold water, rose water and distilled water of the Nile. Regarding the plague, he believed that it was brought into Egypt by contagion from other countries, but that the locals did nothing to prevent it or treat it because of a misguided fatalism.

8.   D. Larrey, *Memoirs of Military Surgery: And Campaigns of the French Armies, on the Rhine, in Corsica, Catalonia, Egypt, and Syria; At Boulogne, Ulm, and Austerlitz; in Saxony, Prussia, Poland, Spain, and Austria / from the French of D. J. Larrey ... by Richard Willmott Hall ... with Notes by the Translator* (Birmingham, AL: Classics of Surgery Library Division of Gryphon Editions, Ltd, 1985), p. 120: 'The English ... followed the method of treatment [for ophthalmia] advised in my memoir, which they found in our hospital in Rosetta', p. 397.

9.   G. Blane, 'To the Editors of the Medical and Physical Journal', *Medical and Physical Journal*, 6 (1801), p. 357.

10. Larrey, *Memoirs*, pp. 397–8.

11. Wilson, *History of the British Expedition to Egypt*, pp. 252–62. In particular, Wilson strongly supports the anti-contagionism of the French regarding plague.

12. Ackerknecht, *Medicine at the Paris Hospital*.

13. Ibid., pp. 25, 37.

14. R. Desgenettes, 'Circular Letter, from Citizen Desgenettes, to the Medical Men of the Army of the East, Relative to a Plan for Drawing up a Physico-Medical Topography of Egypt', in Anon., *Memoirs Relative to Egypt, Written in that Country during the Campaigns of General Bonaparte, in the Years 1798 and 1799, by the Learned and Scientific Men who Accompanied the French Expedition* (London: T. Gillet for R. Phillips, 1800), p. 67.

15. R. Desgenettes, *Histoire médicale de l'armee d'orient, par le medecin en chief R. Desgenettes* (Paris: Croullebois & Bossange, 1802).

16. Two modern works have been heavily based on Larrey's *Memoirs* and provide some additional commentary on French military medicine: Richardson, *Larrey*; and J. H. Dible, *Napoleon's Surgeon* (London: Heinemann Medical, 1970).

17. Larrey, *Memoirs*, p. 156.

18. Ibid., p. 157.

19. Richardson, *Larrey*, p. 62. Richardson gives no reference for this claim.

20. Larrey, *Memoirs*, p. 169.

21. Ibid., p. 193.

22. See the painting commemorating this event by Antoine-Jean Gros, *Napoleon Bonaparte Visiting the Plague-Stricken in Jaffa* (1804).

23. Desgenettes, *Histoire médicale*, pp. 88–9.
24. 'The disease is clearly contagious; but the conditions by which it is transmitted are no more precisely known than its specific nature', Desgenettes, *Histoire médicale*, p. 248; c.f. Ackerknecht, *Medicine at the Paris Hospital*, p. 157: 'The complete sincerity of the anticontagionists was evident in the long series of experiments they undertook on themselves, beginning with Desgenettes' famous plague inoculation in 1798'; and p. 159: 'Desgenettes and Assalini had concluded during Napoleon's expedition that the Egyptian Plague was not contagious'.
25. 'To reassure the shaken imaginations and courage of the army', Desgenettes, *Histoire médicale*, p. 88.
26. P. Assalini, *Observations on the Disease Called the Plague, on the Dysentery, the Ophthalmy of Egypt, and on the Means of Prevention with some Remarks on the Yellow Fever of Cadiz, and the Description and Plan of an Hospital for the Reception of Patients Affected with Epidemic and Contagious Diseases. Translated from the French by Adam Neale of the University of Edinburgh, Member of the Royal College of Surgeons of that City, and Late Surgeon of the Shropshire Regiment of Militia* (New York: T. & J. Swords, 1806), p. 17.
27. A. Jabartî, *Napoleon in Egypt: Al-Jabartî's Chronicle of the French Occupation, 1798*, trans. Shmuel Moreh (Princeton, NJ, and New York: M. Wiener, 1995), pp. 71, 81; on anticontagionism in the French army during this period, and the importance attached to fear as a cause of the disease, see E. A. Heaman, 'The Rise and Fall of Anticontagionism in France', *Canadian Bulletin of Medical History*, 12 (1995), pp. 3–25, on pp. 5–8.
28. Larrey, *Memoirs*, p. 188.
29. Coffee is recommended by nearly every French writer for most diseases encountered in Egypt.
30. Larrey, *Memoirs*, pp. 168–70: 'To the Surgeons of the Army, 22 March 1799'; See also Desgenettes, *Histoire médicale*, pp. 91, 246; Assalini, *Observations*, p. 41. The ill effects of the south wind were formerly identified by Alpinus, *La médicine des Egyptiens*, p. 54.
31. A. Savaresi, 'Essai sur la topographie physique et médicale de Daimiette, suivi d'observations sur les maladies qui ont régné dans cette place, pendant le premiere semester de l'an VII, par le citoyen Savaresi, médecin ordinaire de l'armée', in Desgenettes, *Histoire médicale*, p. 86.
32. Assalini, *Observations*, p. 46; R. Desgenettes, 'Notice Sur l'emploi de l'huile dans la peste', in Desgenettes, *Histoire médicale*, pp. 36–42.
33. Assalini, *Observations*, p. 44
34. Ibid., p. 91.
35. W. Wittman, *Travels in Turkey, Asia-Minor, Syria and Across the Desert into Egypt during the Years 1799, 1800, and 1801, in Company with the Turkish Army, and the British Military Mission. To which are Annexed, Observations on the Plague, and on the Diseases Prevalent in Turkey, and a Meteorological Journal* (London: T. Gillet, 1803).
36. The Egyptian ophthalmia is now thought to have been 'caused by Haemophilus aegyptius, N. gonorrhoea and possibly to some extent by Chlamydia trachomatis but more likely by the adenoviruses'. M. Wagemans and O. van Bijsterveld, 'The French Egyptian Campaign and its Effects on Ophthalmology', *Documenta Ophthalmologica*, 68 (1988), pp. 135–44, on p. 135.
37. '[T]he nitrous particles which continually irritate and inflame the eyes of the inhabitants'. Alpinus, *La médicine des Egyptiens*, p. 93.
38. Savaresi, 'Description et traitement de l'optalmie d'Egypte, par le citoyen Savaresi, médecin ordinaire d'armée d'orient', in Desgenettes, *Histoire médicale*, p. 91. His research

was used by some malingering British and French soldiers to replicate the symptoms of ophthalmia (usually only in one eye).

39. For detailed discussions of the nature, popularity and influence of Brunonianism see W. F. Bynum and R. Porter (eds), *Brunonianism in Britain and Europe* (London: Wellcome Institute for the History of Medicine, 1988); for its influence at the Edinburgh medical schools see, Rosner, *Medical Education in the Age of Improvement*, pp. 129–33.

40. Savaresi, 'Description', pp. 96–9.

41. Bruant, 'Account of the prevailing ophthalmia of Egypt, by citizen Bruant, physician in ordinary to the army, head quarters at Cairo, 15th Fructidor, 6th Year', in Anon., *Memoirs Relative to Egypt*, pp. 110–18.

42. Assalini, *Observations*, pp. 116–53.

43. Larrey, *Memoirs*, p. 113.

44. Ibid.

45. Ibid., p.115.

46. Ibid., p. 109.

47. Desgenettes, *Histoire*, pp. 16, 18, 115.

48. See Cantlie, *A History médicale*, p. 268.

49. For further discussion of Franck see Chapter 4; see also Peterkin et al., *Commissioned Officers*, p. 84.

50. J. McGrigor, *Medical Sketches of the Expedition from Egypt to India* (London: John Murray, 1804), p. 2.

51. Ibid., pp. 94–5.

52. J. McGrigor, 'A Memoir on the State of Health of the 88th Regiment, and of the Corps Attached to it, from 1st June 1800 to the 31st May 1801, as Originally Presented to the Medical Board, Bombay', *EMSJ*, 1 (1805), pp. 266–89.

53. Blanco, *Wellington's Surgeon General*, p. 83.

54. McGrigor, *Medical Sketches*, p. 99.

55. Ibid., pp. 202–17.

56. McGrigor, *Sir James McGrigor. The Scalpel and the Sword*, p. 89.

57. McGrigor, 'A Memoir', p. 285.

58. N. Bruce, 'Remarks on the Dracunculus, or Guinea Worm, as it Appeared in the Peninsula of India', *EMSJ*, 2 (1806), pp. 145–50.

59. An amusing account of this discovery is provided by E. Bancroft in his *An Exposure and Refutation*, 'Dr. McGrigor is very unwilling to admit that a sensation like dismay was excited in any of the medical officers ... However true this observation might prove in the case supposed, I cannot discover that it is applicable to the case of Dr. McGrigor ... for though I did see alarm depicted upon his countenance, and heard several expressions of concern, apparently very sincere, on my announcing to him the state of his two black servants, I have no recollection that those expressions related in any respect to the pitiable condition of his patients, or to any thing but *himself*: all that I remember him to have then expressed, as we left the room ... was, that he felt very unwell, that his legs were so feeble as to be scarcely able to support him ... and that he had great pain in the upper part of one thigh, near the groin (which is the common seat of the pestilential tumors called buboes) ... as soon as we had reached Dr. Shapter's, Dr. McGrigor said he was exhausted and ill, and told a servant to bring him some wine and water', pp. 59–66.

60. McGrigor, *Medical Sketches*, p. 100; P. Russell, *A Treatise of the Plague Containing an Historical Journal and Medical Account of the Plague at Aleppo, in the years 1760, 1761 and 1762* (London: G. G. J. and J. Robinson, 1791).

61. McGrigor, *Medical Sketches*, pp. 143–6.

62. Ibid., p. 41.
63. Ibid., p. 140.
64. Ibid., p. x.
65. Ibid., p. 109.
66. Ibid., p. 56–7.
67. Blanco, *Wellington's Surgeon General*, p. 63.
68. McGrigor, *Medical Sketches*, pp. 140, 237.
69. Ibid., p. 142.
70. Ibid., p. 140. However, it is interesting to contrast this position with the methods McGrigor came to advocate for the treatment of the ophthalmia in Britain, which are discussed later in this chapter.
71. Ibid., p. 141.
72. Ibid., p. 149. 'I believe that several diseases are contagious, which are not suspected to arise from such a cause: the theory of contagion is but very imperfectly understood'.
73. Ibid., p. 159.
74. Ibid., p. 141.
75. H. Dewar, *Observations on Diarrhoea and Dysentery, Particularly as these Diseases Appeared in the British Campaign of Egypt in 1801* (London: John Murray, 1805), p. 119.
76. Wittman, *Travels*, p. 518.
77. McGrigor, *Medical Sketches*, pp. 158–9.
78. Ibid., pp. 137–9.
79. Ibid., p. 104; see also p. 142.
80. Ibid., p. 159.
81. Ibid., p. 15.
82. Ibid., pp. 21, 23.
83. See, Rosner, *Medical Education in the Age of Improvement*, p. 50.
84. Antiphlogistic regimes were designed to reduce inflammation. During the early nineteenth century practitioners in the tropics, including Robert Jackson, promoted therapeutic regimes focused on reducing inflammation, principally through bleeding. Mercurials were sometimes used by these practitioners as purgatives alongside bloodletting, see P. Niebyl, 'The English Bloodletting Revolution, or Modern Medicine before 1850', *Bulletin of the History of Medicine*, 51 (1977), pp. 472–4. As already noted, Jackson had a great influence on military therapeutics, and the increasing incidence of this type of generally antiphlogistic regime among military practitioners at this time is further evidence of this point. Similar ideas were advanced by the French military practitioner François Broussais, see: E. H. Ackerknecht, 'Broussais, or A Forgotten Medical Revolution', *Bulletin of the History of Medicine*, 27 (1953), pp. 320–43.
85. McGrigor, *Medical Sketches*, pp. 146–59.
86. H. Dewar, *Dissertatio medica inauguralis, de ophthalmia Ægypti: quam ... pro gradu doctoris ...* (Edinburgh: Creech, 1804).
87. Dewar, *Observations*, p. 36.
88. D. Whyte, 'Mode of Managing Ocular Inflammations', *Medical and Physical Journal*, 7 (1802), pp. 209–16.
89. G. Power, *Attempt to Investigate the Cause of Egyptian Ophthalmia, with Observations on its Nature and Different Modes of Cure* (London: John Murray, 1803).
90. Ibid., pp. 10–14.
91. Ibid., p. 19.
92. Ibid., pp. 21.

93. Ibid., pp. 22–4.
94. Ibid., p. 61.
95. Ibid., p. 63.
96. McGrigor, *Medical Sketches*, pp. 181–2.
97. Ibid., pp. 182–3.
98. Dewar, *Observations*, p. 71.
99. Ibid., pp. 111–19.
100. Ibid., p. 92.
101. Ibid., pp. 5–6, 29.
102. McGrigor, *Medical Sketches*, p. 68.
103. McGrigor, 'A Memoir', p. 266.
104. McGrigor, *Medical Sketches*, p. 5; see also, for example, reviews of many of these works: S. Hall, 'Some Account of a Recent French Publication, Respecting the Pestilential and Malignant Fevers of the Levant', *Medical and Physical Journal*, 8 (1802), pp. 449–53; 'A Description of the Egyptian Ophthalmia, and the Method of Treatment. By Cit. Savaresi, Physician in ordinary to the (French) Army of the East', *Medical and Physical Journal*, 8 (1802), pp. 555–8; 'Relation historique et chirurgicale de l'expedition de l'armee s'orient, en Egypte et en Syrie. Par D. J. Larrey, docteur de l'ecole speciale de medicine de Paris; chirurgien en chef de l'armee d'orient, &c. &c. 8vo Paris 1804', *EMSJ*, 2 (1806), pp. 213–23.
105. For an account of the return to Britain of the troops and accompanying incidences of ophthalmia see M. Meyerhof, 'A Short History of Ophthalmia during the Egyptian Campaigns of 1798–1807', *British Journal of Ophthalmology*, 16 (1932), pp. 138–47; for ophthalmia in the Prussian Army see Hirschberg, *The History*, p. 295; for the Belgian Army see G. Gorin, *History of Ophthalmology* (Delaware: Publish or Perish, 1982), p. 92.
106. McGrigor was quick to identify the disease as the same as the one which had prevailed in Egypt: 'McGrigor to Knight', 8 August 1806, WL, RAMC 799, McGrigor Correspondence Book 1. The rising numbers of ophthalmic cases amongst the troops is well documented in McGrigor's letters to Knight throughout this volume and the following Correspondence Book 2.
107. 'A Treatise on the Varieties and Consequences of Ophthalmia, with a Preliminary Inquiry into its Contagious Nature. By Arthur Edmondston, M. D. Fellow of the Royal College of Surgeons, and Honorary Member of the Royal Physical Society of Edinburgh. Edinburgh, 1806. 8vo. Pp.319', *EMSJ*, 3 (1807), p. 211.
108. A. Edmonston, *A Treatise on the Varieties and Consequences of Ophthalmia with a Preliminary Inquiry into its Contagious Nature* (Edinburgh: W. Blackwood, 1806), p. 31.
109. Ibid., pp. 37–8.
110. Ibid., p. 31.
111. Ibid., p. 98.
112. Ibid., p. 12; see also P. MacGregor, 'An account of an ophthalmia which prevailed in the Royal Military Asylum, in 1804. By Patrick MacGregor, Esq. surgeon to the Royal Military Asylum, and assistant surgeon to the lock hospital, read April 2, 1805', *Transactions of a Society for the Improvement of Medical and Chirurgical Knowledge* 3 (1812), pp. 30–44.
113. Edmonston, *A Treatise*, pp. 38–45; see also, Anon., *Identities Ascertained or, An Illustration of Mr Ware's Opinion Respecting the Sameness of Infection in Venereal Gonorrhaea, and the Ophthalmia of Egypt: With an Examination of Affinity between Antient Leprosy and Lues* (London: J. & W. Smith, 1808), pp. 17–40.

114. Edmonston, *A Treatise*, p. 225.
115. J. Vetch, *An Account of the Ophthalmia which has Appeared in England since the Return of the British Army from Egypt* (London, 1807), p. iv.
116. Ibid., p. 69.
117. Ibid., p. 6–14
118. Ibid., p. 15.
119. Ibid., p. 19.
120. Ibid., pp. 84–92
121. Ibid., p. 95.
122. Ibid., p. 97.
123. 'An Account of the Ophthalmia which has Appeared in England, since the Return of the British Army from Egypt. By John Vetch, M.D. Member of the Medical Society of Edinburgh, and Assistant Surgeon to the 54th Foot. London. 1807. 8vo. pp.142', *EMSJ*, 3 (1807), p. 366.
124. Vetch, *An Account*, p. 127; similar advice had been given the previous year in a circular from the adjutant general's office to generals commanding districts, TNA, WO 123/134, p. 545: 23 September 1806.
125. 'Observations on the Epidemic Ophthalmia, as it Affected the Troops in Hythe Barracks. In a Letter from George Peach, Esq. Surgeon of the 2d Battalion 52nd Foot, at Reading-Street Barracks, Kent, to James McGrigor, M.D. Deputy Inspector-General of Hospitals, Portsmouth', *EMSJ*, 3 (1807), pp. 52–5.
126. Ibid., p. 54.
127. J. Ware, *Remarks on the Purulent Ophthalmy, which has Lately been Epidemical in this Country* (London: J. Mawman, 1808), p. 25.
128. 'Observations on the Epidemic Ophthalmia, as it Affected the Troops in Hythe Barracks', p. 55.
129. Ibid.
130. 'Further Observations on the Egyptian Ophthalmia, as it Affected the 2nd Battalion of the 52nd Regiment. In a Letter from George Peach, Esq. Surgeon to the 2nd Battalion 52nd Regiment, to James M'Gregor, M.D. Fellow of the Royal College of Physicians, Edinburgh, and Deputy Inspector-General of Hospitals, Portsmouth', *EMSJ*, 3 (1807), pp. 395–400.
131. Ibid., p. 396.
132. 'Egyptian Ophthalmia', *London Medical and Surgical Spectator*, 1 (1808), p. 116.
133. Hirschberg, *A History*, p. 91.
134. C. Farrell, *Observations on Ophthalmia and its Consequences* (London: John Murray, 1811), pp. 69–70.
135. Ibid., p. 55.
136. 'Observations on the History and Treatment of an Epidemic Ophthalmia, which Appeared in the Fourth Battalion of the Royals, in Edinburgh Castle, during the Months of July and August 1807, By C.F. Forbes, Esq. Surgeon of the Royals', *EMSJ*, 3 (1807), pp. 430–4.
137. Ware, *Remarks*, pp. 2, 8.
138. Anon., *Identities Ascertained*, pp. 3–4.
139. 'Surgery', *London Medical and Surgical Spectator*, 2 (1809), p. 143.
140. 'Remarks on the Difference between the Infectious Ophthalmia, and that Produced by the Artful Application of Irritating Substances to the Eyes. By John Vetch, M.D. Assis-

tant Surgeon with Ophthalmia Detachments at Riding Street Barracks', *EMSJ*, 4 (1808), pp. 157–9.

141. Hirschberg, *A History*, p. 76.
142. 'Report from the select committee on the ophthalmic hospital', 3 July 1821, *CCR* (1824), 6:417, p. 337.
143. General Orders, no. 187: 'Report of a Special Medical Board, which has been Assembled to Take into Consideration the Prevalence of the Purulent Ophthalmia in the Army', 5 February 1810, TNA, WO 123/130.

4 The Peninsular War

1. It is not possible to give a detailed military history of the campaigns of the Peninsular War here. A vast body of scholarship on all aspects of the war and the campaigns of the British armies exists, ranging from the weighty and seminal work of C. W. C. Oman, *A History of the Peninsular War* (Oxford: Clarendon Press, 1902–30); to the more accessible works of C. J. Esdaile, *The Peninsular War: A New History* (London: Penguin, 2003); D. Gates, *The Spanish Ulcer, A History of the Peninsular War* (London: Pimlico, 2002); and M. Glover, *The Peninsular War, 1807–1814, A Concise Military History* (London: Penguin, 2001).
2. Principally: Cantlie, *A History*, chs 10, 11; Blanco, *Wellington's Surgeon General*; Glover, *Wellington's Army in the Peninsula 1808–1814*, ch. 10; M. R. Howard, 'Medical Aspects of Sir John Moore's Corunna Campaign, 1808–1809', *Journal of the Royal Society of Medicine*, 84 (1991), pp. 299–302; Howard, *Wellington's Doctors*; Kaufman, *Surgeons at War*, ch. 2; G. Kempthorne, 'The Medical Department of Wellington's Army, 1809–1814', *Journal of the Royal Army Medical Corps*, 54 (1930), pp. 65–72, 131–46, 212–19; and J. Watts, 'George James Guthrie, Peninsular Surgeon', *Proceedings of the Royal Society of Medicine* (1961), pp. 764–8.
3. McGrigor, *Sir James McGrigor. The Scalpel and the Sword*, chs 13–18; J. McGrigor, 'Sketch of the Medical History of the British Armies in the Peninsula of Spain and Portugal during the Late Campaigns', *Medico-Chirurgical Transactions*, 6 (1815), pp. 381–488.
4. A typical account of Guthrie's heroics (both surgical and otherwise) can be found in Watts, 'George James Guthrie', especially p. 765.
5. Cantlie, *A History*, p. 338.
6. Blanco, *Wellington's Surgeon General*, p. 118
7. See Cantlie, *A History*, pp. 320–2; Kaufman, *Surgeons at War*, p. 76; Rosner, *The Most Beautiful Man*, pp. 110–13.
8. For a detailed history of the retreat, see C. Hibbert, *Corunna* (Moreton-In-Marsh: Windrush, 1996).
9. A. Neale, *Letters from Portugal and Spain; Comprising an Account of the Operations of the Armies under their Excellencies Sir Arthur Wellesley and Sir John Moore, from the Landing of the Troops in Mondego Bay to the Battle at Corunna* (London: T. Gillet, 1809), pp. 304–5.
10. Ibid., pp. 276–9.
11. Ibid., p. 284.
12. This opinion was shared by McGrigor, who further stated that the Marquis de Romana's army had contracted the fever in the Baltic, J. McGrigor, 'Observations on the Fever

which Appeared in the Army from Spain on their Return to this Country in January 1809', *EMSJ*, 6 (1810), pp. 19–32, on p. 19.

13. Anon., 'Journal of a Soldier of the LXXI Regiment from 1806 to 1815', in *Constable's Miscellany of Original and Selected Publications in the Various Departments of Literature, Science and the Arts* (Edinburgh, 1828), vol. 27, p. 69.

14. 'Letter from AMB to J. Pultney', 23 January 1809, TNA, WO 4/407, p. 76.

15. Kaufman, *Surgeons at War*, p. 62.

16. McGrigor, 'Observations on the Fever', p. 19.

17. 'Dent to his Mother', 17 February 1809, WL, RAMC 536, Dent Letters, f. 4.

18. 'Dent to his Mother', 5 March 1809, WL, RAMC 536, Dent Letters, f. 5.

19. 'Dent to his Mother', 7 May 1810, WL, RAMC 536, Dent Letters, f. 13; 'Dent to his Mother', 21 May 1810, WL, RAMC 536, Dent Letters, f. 14.

20. 'Dent to his Mother', 24 June 1810, WL, RAMC 536, Dent Letters, f. 15.

21. 'Dent to his Mother', 22 April 1810, WL, RAMC 536, Dent Letters, f. 12.

22. 'John Murray to his father', 17 August 1809, WL, RAMC 830, Murray letters: 'on actual service the Surgeons and medical men have the finest field for information open to them in the space of on single month they perhaps see more and get more experience (if they pay attention) than a man in private practice may, during his whole life time'; R. Gibney (ed.), *Eighty Years Ago, or the Recollections of an Old Army Doctor, His Adventures on the Field of Quatre Bras and Waterloo and during the Occupation of Paris in 1815, by the Late Dr. Gibney of Cheltenham* (London: Bellairs & Company, 1896), p. 92.

23. It is not suggested that this belief in the value of 'on-the-field' experience was advocated to the absolute exclusion of formal study; consider the experience of a practitioner who had undertaken a much more formal education before entering the army medical service who was told on his examination that although his answers were 'book perfect', he would soon learn that 'on-the-field of battle' would prove to be a more valuable learning experience than traditional book-learning. Gibney (ed.), *Eighty Years Ago*, p. 92.

24. R. Hooper, 'Account of the Diseases of the Sick Landed at Plymouth from Corunna', *EMSJ*, 5 (1809), pp. 398–420.

25. Ibid., p. 400.

26. Ibid., p. 401.

27. McGrigor, 'Observations on the Fever', p. 27.

28. The effect of hierarchical military structures in the production of a uniform approach to medical practice is discussed by Harrison in, 'Disease and Medicine in the Armies of British India', pp. 95, 104–6.

29. McGrigor, 'Observations on the Fever', p. 26.

30. Ibid., p. 20.

31. Ibid., p. 22.

32. 'Pepys and Keate to Pultney', 14 April 1809, TNA, WO 1/641, f. 15.

33. 'Neale to Pepys', 6 April 1809, TNA, WO 1/641, ff. 19–25. Neale was a great advocate of general hospitals: 'In spite of all the silly clamour which has lately been raised against the great establishment of general hospitals, their utility is great, and with men on service, undeniable. The French attempted to do without them at the beginning of the last war, but the experiment failed.' Neale, *Letters*, p. 38.

34. 'Tice to Pepys', 8 April 1809, TNA, WO 1/641, ff. 27–9.

35. 'Faulkner to Pepys', 14 April 1809, TNA, WO 1/641, ff. 39–42.

36. 'Edward Knight to Pepys', 28 March 1809, TNA, WO 1/641, ff. 43–35.

37. 'Dundas to Castlereagh', 23 June 1809, TNA, WO 1/641, f. 184.

38. 'Knight to Moore', 18 April 1809, TNA, WO 1/641, f. 31–33.
39. 'Dundas to Castlereagh', 23 June 1809, TNA, WO 1/641, f. 184.
40. 'Report of board of general officers', 20 June 1809, TNA, WO 1/641, ff. 185–207.
41. Ibid., ff. 191–2.
42. Ibid., f. 200.
43. Ibid., f. 203.
44. Ibid., f. 205.
45. 'Gower to Pepys and Keate', 12 July 1809, TNA, WO 1/237, p. 26.
46. T. Catherwood, 'A Narrative of some of the Transactions of the Purveyors Department, which Served with the Army in the Peninsula under the Command of the Duke of Wellington, with Anecdotes Relative to the Conduct of the Medical Department of the Army', WL, MS 1529, p. 12.
47. Blanco, *Wellington's Surgeon General*, p. 111.
48. Cantlie provides extensive detail on the arrangements that were made to convey soldiers from the frontline and the regimental hospitals to the general hospitals that were established in major towns at the rear. He explains how the scarcity of transport meant that the 'accepted practice' of treating the sick and wounded in regimental hospitals had to be abandoned because there were not enough transports to convey all the wounded with the army as it moved. Wellesley also believed that conveying the wounded with the army would impede his ability to move quickly, *A History*, p. 310. On transport difficulties generally see, Cantlie, *A History*, ch. 10. More detailed accounts of these campaigns can also be found in Kaufman, *Surgeons at War*, ch. 2; and Glover, *The Peninsular War*, part 3.
49. 3,915 (1,448 killed), Cantlie, *A History*, p. 314.
50. For an account of Guthrie's efforts, see Cantlie, *A History*, pp. 314–16.
51. Cantlie, *A History*, p. 317; see also E. Costello, *The Adventures of a Soldier; Or Memoirs of Edward Costello K.S.F., Formerly a Non-Commissioned Officer in the Rifle Brigade, and Late Captain in the British Legion* (London: Henry Colburn, 1841), p. 36: 'we remained here three months, during which time a dreadful mortality took place. In our regiment, alone, the flux and brain fever reigned to so frightful an extent, that *three hundred* men died in hospital'. Costello also describes the prevailing treatment for the disease at the hospital in Elvas: 'it principally consisted in throwing cold water from canteens or mess kettles as often as possible over the bodies of the patients; this in many cases was effectual, and I think cured me', p. 37; see also J. Sherer, *Recollections of the Peninsula, by the Author of Sketches of India*, 2nd edn (London: Longman et al., 1824), p. 72: 'this insidious and resistless enemy found his way into our tranquil quarters, crowded our hospitals with sick, and filled the chapel vaults with victims, over whom we gloomily and sullenly mourned'.
52. For a first-hand description of the sufferings of the wounded see Sherer, *Recollections*, pp. 153–65.
53. 'Wellington to Liverpool', TNA, WO 1/242, pp. 287–300; 'Wellington to Liverpool', 29 November 1809, TNA, WO 1/242, p. 445; 'Wellington to Liverpool', 14 December 1809, TNA, WO 1/242, p. 549.
54. 'Garrison Orders', 24 August 1810, TNA, WO 134/3.
55. 'Garrison Orders', 29 August 1810, TNA, WO 134/3.
56. 'AMB to Franck', 22 December 1810, TNA, WO 7/109, p. 19.
57. 'AMB to Franck', 10 February 1811, TNA, WO 7/109, p. 68.
58. 'AMB to Franck', 22 December 1810, TNA, WO 7/109, p. 20.

59. 'General Orders, Pero Negro', 23 October 1810, TNA, WO 134/2. The reluctance of convalescent officers to leave Lisbon is perhaps explained by Sherer's account of his time there: 'At Libson, the period of my convalescence glided away with the most pleasing rapidity. I dined daily in a most agreeable society; I passed my mornings in studying the Portuguese and Spanish languages; and oftentimes, of an evening, muffled up as an invalid, I stole in a cabriolet, to the theatre of San Carlos, or the Opera Buffa', *Recollections*, p. 81.

60. 'AMB to Franck', 21 February 1811, TNA, WO 7/109, p. 73. For similar evidence of Franck and Borland's resentment of the AMB's supervision of their practice see: 'AMB to Franck', 22 January 1811, TNA, WO 7/109, pp. 43–5; 'AMB to Franck', 29 July 1811, TNA, WO 7/109, p. 141; 'AMB to Bolton', 20 September 1811, TNA, WO 7/109, p. 161.

61. 'AMB to Franck', 29 July 1811, TNA, WO 7/109, p. 141.

62. 'AMB to Borland', 24 September 1811, TNA, WO 7/109, p. 162.

63. Ibid., p. 166.

64. 'General Orders, Quinta de Banos', 7 July 1811, TNA, WO 134/3.

65. 'AMB to Franck', 8 January 1811, TNA, WO 7/109, p. 32.

66. Ibid.

67. Ibid., p. 33; see also, 'AMB to Fellows', 8 January 1811, TNA, WO 7/109, p. 38.

68. 'AMB to Franck', 8 March 1811, TNA, WO 7/109, p. 77, my emphasis.

69. 'AMB to Fellows', 19 November 1810, TNA, WO 7/109, p. 6.

70. 'AMB to Fellows', 29 November 1810, TNA, WO 7/109, pp. 11–12.

71. 'AMB to Franck', 9 July 1811, TNA, WO 7109, p. 134.

72. 'AMB to Franck', 22 December 1810, TNA, WO 7/109, p. 21.

73. 'AMB to Franck', 7 January 1811, TNA, WO 7/109, p. 37.

74. 'AMB to Franck', 10 February 1811, TNA, WO 7/109, pp. 67–8.

75. Quoted in Kempthorne, 'The Medical Department of Wellington's Army, 1809–1814', pp. 145–6. Kempthorne gives no reference for this quotation. Kempthorne is referenced by Cantlie, Blanco, and Kaufman in the repetition of this story.

76. 'AMB to McGrigor', 31 March 1812, TNA, WO 7/109, p. 238; 'AMB to McGrigor', 6 April 1812, TNA, WO 7/109, p. 240.

77. A brief account of the British surgeons who served with the Portuguese Army can be found in M. Giao, 'British Surgeons in the Portuguese Army during the Peninsular War', *Journal of the Royal Army Medical Corps*, 62 (1934), pp. 298–303.

78. Short descriptions of Fergusson's reforms are included in Cantlie, *A History*, pp. 320–2; Kaufman, *Surgeons at War*, p. 76–7; Rosner, *The Most Beautiful Man*, ch. 8.

79. Fergusson, *William Fergusson, Notes and Recollections*, pp. xii–xiii; see also C. Charles, 'Fergusson, William (1773–1846)', rev. J. Reznick, *ODNB*, online at http://www.oxforddnb.com/view/article/9339 [accessed 23 January 2008].

80. Fergusson, *William Fergusson, Notes and Recollections*; William Fergusson papers, WL, RAMC 208–12.

81. 'Proceedings of a general court martial held on William Pitt Munston of the Royal South Lincoln Militia', 22 October 1807, WL, RAMC 212, p. 41.

82. 'Regimental Hospitals – Preliminary Observations', WL, RAMC 210.3.

83. 'Knight to Fergusson', 13 August 1806, WL, RAMC 212, p. 61.

84. Rosner, *The Most Beautiful Man*, pp. 76, 97.

85. Neale, *Letters*, p. 38.

86. The database used to compile data for Ackroyd et al., *Advancing with the Army*, reveals that Ross graduated MA from Marischal College in 1785, and obtained the RCS diploma in London in 1803 (database doctor identity number 397). Ross had previously been reprimanded by Sir James Pultney for writing about his superior officer (Fergusson) in language that 'was not sufficiently respectful', in 'Moore to Ross', 3 May 1809, TNA, WO 4/407, p. 360.
87. 'Ross to Wellesley', 5 June 1809, WL, RAMC 211.2, pp. 13–15.
88. 'Moore to Gordon', 31 January 1809, TNA, WO 4/407, p. 95: 'Having ... called upon the Principal Officers of the AMD to state the objections they alluded to in regard to Dr. Jackson'.
89. 10 June 1809, WL, RAMC 211.2, pp. 16–17.
90. See for example, 'W. Wallace to Fergusson', 11 June 1809, WL, RAMC 211.2, pp. 18–19; (and, in the same record) 'Burminster to Fergusson', 11 June 1809, p. 20; 'Beacham to Fergusson', 11 June 1809, pp. 21–2; 'Guthrie to Fergusson', 11 June 1809, pp. 24–7; 'Cook to Fergusson', 12 June 1809, pp. 22–4; 'Bell to Fergusson', 15 June 1809, p. 30; 'Irwin to Fergusson', 15 June 1809, pp. 31–2; 'Forbes to Fergusson', 15 June 1809, p. 33; 'Mackey to Fergusson', 15 June 1809, pp. 34–5; 'Gunning to Fergusson', 16 June 1809, pp. 34–6; 'Kidd to Fergusson', 18 June 1809, p. 36.
91. 'Moore to Surgeon General', 22 July 1809, TNA, WO 4/408, p. 69; 'Moore to Surgeon General', 8 August 1809, TNA, WO 4/408, p. 116.
92. 'Moore to Inspector General of Army Hospitals', 15 April 1809, TNA, WO 4/407, p. 299.
93. McGrigor, *Sir James McGrigor. The Scalpel and the Sword*, p. 164.
94. Ibid., p. 164. However, see 'Moore to Torrens', 21 November 1809, TNA, WO 4/409, p. 43, enclosing 'Mr Knights report, recommending ... Dy Inspector Wm Fergusson'.
95. The number of staff surgeons was later increased to twenty.
96. A. Halliday, *Observations on the Present State of the Portuguese Army, As Organised by Lieutenant-General Sir William Carr Beresford, K. B. Field Marshall and Commander in Chief of that Army. With an Account of the Different Military Establishments and Laws of Portugal, and a Sketch of the Campaigns of the Last and Present Year, during which the Portuguese Army was Brought into the Field Against the Enemy, for the First Time as a Regular Force* (London: John Murray, 1811), p. 87.
97. Ibid., p. 87.
98. Accordingly, the accounts of the Portuguese Medical Service by British medical officers included here are intended to illustrate British opinions and how the environment in which those men found themselves contributed to the production of a professional identity, not the actual state of Portuguese military medicine during this period.
99. Halliday, *Observations on the Present State of the Portugese Army*, p. 93.
100. A. Schaumann, *On the Road with Wellington, The Diary of a War Commissary in the Peninsular Campaigns*, ed. and trans. A. M. Ludovici (London: W. Heinemann, 1924), p. 222.
101. S. Broughton, *Letters from Portugal, Spain and France* (1815; Stroud: Nonsuch, 2005), p. 64.
102. Halliday, *Observations*, p. 83
103. Ibid.
104. Ibid., p. 84.
105. Ibid., p. 85.
106. Ibid.

107. 'Thomas to Keate', 10 November 1809, WL, RAMC 208.3, p. 223.

108. 'Wynn to Fergusson', 11 February 1810, WL, RAMC 208.3, p. 271; and in the same record: 'Jebb to Fergusson', 13 February 1810, p. 111; 'Thomas to Fergusson', 15 February 1810, p. 227; 'Griffith to Fergusson', 15 February 1810, p. 55; 'West to Fergusson', 6 March 1810, p. 251; 'Halliday to Fergusson', 8 March 1810, p. 99.

109. 'Thomas to Fergusson', 8 June 1810, WL, RAMC 212, p. 50.

110. For example, 'Wynn to Fergusson', WL, RAMC 212, p. 67: 'Do you not think, in general, and particularly in the field, that surgeons are more useful being competent to the duty of physician as well as their own? An additional deputy Inspector would probably be of more real use than half a dozen physicians.'

111. 'Jebb to Fergusson', 13 February 1810, WL, RAMC 208.3, p. 111.

112. 'Fergusson to D'Urban', 7 May 1810, WL, RAMC 208.2, p. 21–2.

113. 'Fergusson to Robertson', 16 May 1810, WL, RAMC 208.3, p. 191.

114. 'Robertson to Fergusson', 19 June 1810, WL, RAMC 212, p. 17.

115. 'Fergusson to Arbuthnot', 5 September 1810, WL, RAMC 208.5, p. 43.

116. 'Weir to Fergusson', 23 October 1810, WL, RAMC 208.5, p. 83.

117. 'Blunt to Fergusson', 5 September 1810, WL, RAMC 208.3, p. 5.

118. 'Arbuthnot to Fergusson', 23 November 1810, WL, RAMC 212, p. 38.

119. 'Blunt to Fergusson', 5 September 1810, WL, RAMC 208.3, p. 5; 'Blunt to Fergusson', 15 November 1810, WL, RAMC 212, p. 70; 'Blunt to Fergusson', 5 December 1810, WL, RAMC 208.3, pp. 13–15; 'Blunt to Fergusson', 22 December 1810, WL, RAMC 212, p. 72.

120. 'Blunt to Fergusson', 15 November 1810, RAMC 212, p. 70.

121. Fergusson, *William Fergusson, Notes and Recollections*, p. 67.

122. Ibid.

123. 'Fergusson to Frank', 23 May 1811, WL, RAMC 210, p. 1.

124. J. Gurwood, *The General Orders of Field Marshal the Duke of Wellington K. D. &c. &c .&c. in Portugal, Spain, and France, from 1809 to 1814; and the Low Countries and France, 1815* (London: Clowes & Sons, 1832), p. 217: 'Portuguese Authorities', *Freneda*, 7 December 1811.

125. 'Fergusson to Hardinge', 26 June 1811, WL, RAMC 210.1, p. 13.

126. 'A plan submitted to His Excellency Sir William Carr Berefsord Marshal Commander in Chief of the Portuguese forces for the regulation of its medical department', WL, RAMC 210.1, p. 21; see also WL, RAMC 210.3.

127. 'Jebb to Fergusson', 4 October 1811, WL, RAMC 208.3, p. 123; 'Morse to Fergusson', 11 October 1811, WL, RAMC 212, p. 88; 'Fergusson to D'Urban', 15 November 1811, WL, RAMC 210.1, pp. 74–8.

128. 'Fergusson to Arbuthnot', 16 December 1811, WL, RAMC, 210.1.

129. 'Griffith to Fergusson', 23 January 1812, WL, RAMC, 208.3, p. 75.

130. 'Morse to Fergusson', 20 January 1812, WL, RAMC, 208.3, p. 167.

131. 'Fergusson to Arbuthnot', 3 February 1812, WL, RAMC, 210.1, p. 82–6.

132. 'Arbuthnot to Fergusson', 29 February 1812, WL, RAMC 208.2, p.111–13.

133. 'McGrigor to AMB', 29 April 1812, WL, RAMC 799.6, p. 8.

134. J. Gurwood, *The Dispatches of Field Marshal the Duke of Wellington: During his Various Campaigns in India, Denmark, Portugal, Spain, the Low Countries, and France, from 1799 to 1818*, 13 vols (London: John Murray, 1838), vol. 7, p. 174.

135. 'Callendar to Fergusson', 1 March 1812, WL, RAMC 208.3, p. 29.

136. 'Griffith to Fergusson', 5 March, 1812, WL, RAMC 208.3, p. 79–82.

137. 'Murray to his brother', 6 July 1812, WL, RAMC 830, Murray Letters.
138. 'M. Fergusson to Fergusson', 17 March 1812, WL, RAMC 208.3, p. 161; On Fergusson's efforts, and the inutility of his patrons for this purpose, see Ackroyd et al., *Advancing with the Army*, p. 200. Ackroyd et al. also suggest that Fergusson had been quarrelling with Beresford over the deployment of regimental hospitals.
139. 'Kindell to Fergusson', 2 March 1812, WL, RAMC 208.3, p. 143.
140. 'Fergusson to Blunt', 30 July 1812, WL, RAMC 210.1.
141. Ibid.
142. 'Wynn to Fergusson', 9 August 1812, WL, RAMC 208.2, p. 151.
143. 'Fergusson to Beresford', 1 November 1812, WL, RAMC 210.1.
144. 14 November 1812, WL, RAMC 208.2, p. 169.
145. Fergusson's approach here is one of the best examples of the ways in which military medical officers used language to make claims to their superior officers for their specialized 'military medicine'. These attempts reflect David Harley's observation on the use of rhetoric in medicine: 'The presentation of medical ideas in an open market requires them to connect with the core beliefs of a substantial group of potential patients'. 'Rhetoric and the Social Construction of Sickness and Healing', *Social History of Medicine*, 12 (1999), pp. 407–35, on p. 414.

5 James McGrigor in the Peninsula

1. Cantlie, *A History*, p. 357 (quoting Napier); Blanco, *Wellington's Surgeon General*, pp. 136, 141–2.
2. Blanco, *Wellington's Surgeon General*, p. 137.
3. 'McGrigor to Borland', 19 November 1805, WL, RAMC 799, p. 30.
4. 'Borland to Irwin', 26 November 1805, WL, RAMC 799, pp. 34–5, my emphasis.
5. 'McGrigor to Robinson', 28 May 1806, WL, RAMC 799, p. 58.
6. '[?] to Knight', 22 January 1808, WL, RAMC 799, pp. 223–4.
7. 'McGrigor to Evelegh', 29 February 1808, WL, RAMC 799, (book II), p. 11; see also 'McGrigor to Savary', 2 October 1807, WL, RAMC 799, (book II), p. 177.
8. 'Weir and Kennedy to McGrigor', 5 October 1810, TNA, WO 7/107, p. 39.
9. 'Weir and Kennedy to McGrigor', 3 December 1810, TNA, WO 7/107, p. 125.
10. 'Reed to McGrigor', 18 January 1811, TNA, WO 7/107, p. 165.
11. 'McGrigor to Board', 8 October 1810, see for example, WL, RAMC 799, pp. 131–3.
12. McGrigor, *Sir James McGrigor. The Scalpel and the Sword*, p. 175.
13. Ibid., p. 179.
14. 'Wellington to Liverpool', April 8 1812, TNA, WO 1/254, p. 59.
15. 'McGrigor to Reed', undated, following a letter dated 18 May 1812, WL, RAMC 799/6, p. 27.
16. 'McGrigor to Reed', 25 August 1812, TNA, WO 799/6, p. 101.
17. McGrigor, *Sir James McGrigor. The Scalpel and the Sword*, p. 202.
18. Ibid., p. 207.
19. Ibid., p. 215.
20. Ibid.
21. Ibid., p. 222. After this date, the system of regimental hospitals appears to have become the accepted 'best practice' in the administration of army medical services, see for example, 'Torrens to Bunbury', 6 December 1814, TNA, WO 1/659, p. 571: 'the Commander in Chief has no hesitation in stating it to be his opinion that the system of regimen-

tal Hospitals is most advantageous to the Service, and that His Royal Highness would therefore be inclined to recommend ... that Regimental Hospitals should be erected at Gibraltar in preference to a large General Hospital'.

22. 'McGrigor to Army Medical Board', 13 January 1814, TNA, WO 799/8, p. 148–9.
23. Guthrie, *Commentaries*, p. 146.
24. T. Catherwood, 'Narrative of Events in the Peninsular Campaign, Compiled 1816–18', WL, MS 1529, p. 32; note that a review of the Wellington Papers Database administered by the University of Southampton, online at http://www.archives.soton.ac.uk/ wellington/, reveals nothing that would indicate that McGrigor was the recipient of any special attentions from Wellington after the Wars, other than Wellington's support for McGrigor's application for a Baronetcy.
25. S. G. P. Ward, *Wellington's Headquarters: A Study of the Administrative Problems in the Peninsula, 1809–1814* (London: Oxford University Press, 1957), pp. 39–45, ch. 6.
26. 'AMB to McGrigor', 6 April 1812, TNA, WO 7/109, p. 242. In this thinking the Board may have been influenced by the reduction of typhus fever in the British Navy by this time, and also by the strong associations between typhus fever and a lack of hygiene and discipline. See G. Blane, 'Statements of the Comparative Health of the British Navy, from the Year 1779 to the Year 1814, with Proposals for its Farther Improvement', *Medico-Chirurgical Transactions*, 6 (1815), pp. 490–573, on pp. 503–12.
27. 'AMB to McGrigor', 6 April 1812, TNA, WO 7/109, p. 244.
28. 'AMB to McGrigor', 7 April 1812, TNA, WO 7/109, p. 246.
29. 'Reed to McGrigor', 19 May 1812, TNA, WO 7/109, p. 273–4.
30. 'AMB to McGrigor', 11 May 1812, TNA, WO 7/109, p. 268.
31. 'AMB to McGrigor', 22 May 1812, TNA, WO 7/109, p. 274.
32. Ibid., p. 276.
33. 'McGrigor to Wellington and AMB', 23 May 1812, WL, RAMC 799/6, p. 31.
34. 'McGrigor to Commander of the Forces', 8 June 1812, WL, RAMC 799/6, pp. 39–40.
35. 'Wellington to Liverpool', 12 June 1812, TNA, WO 1/254, p. 635.
36. 'McGrigor to Wellington', 12 June 1812, TNA, WO 1/254, p. 639.
37. 'AMB to McGrigor', 10 July 1812, TNA, WO 7/109, p. 302.
38. 'McGrigor to Reed', 10 August 1812, WL, RAMC 799/6, p. 88.
39. 'McGrigor to Reed', 28 July 1812, WL, RAMC 799/6, p. 74.
40. 'McGrigor to AMB', 28 July 1812, WL, RAMC 799/6, pp. 74–6.
41. 'AMB to McGrigor', 1 September 1812, TNA, WO 7/109, p. 323.
42. 'McGrigor to Reed', 15 July 1812, WL, RAMC 799/6, pp. 64–6.
43. 'McGrigor to Wellington', 24 July 1812, WL, RAMC 799/6, p. 72.
44. 'McGrigor to Weir', 29 April 1812, WL, RAMC 799/6, p. 12.
45. 'Weir to McGrigor', 18 August 1812, TNA, WO 7/109, p. 313.
46. 'McGrigor to Weir', 27 September 1812, WL, RAMC 799/6, p. 123.
47. 'Weir to McGrigor', 2 October 1812, TNA, WO 7/109, p. 345.
48. 'McGrigor to Weir', 27 September 1812, WL, RAMC 799/6, p. 123.
49. 'McGrigor to Reed', 14 May 1812, WL, RAMC 799/6, p. 22; 'McGrigor to AMB', 24 November 1812, WL, RAMC 799/6, p. 156.
50. 'McGrigor to Weir', 26 November 1812, WL, RAMC 799/6, p. 158.
51. 'AMB to McGrigor', 5 October 1812, TNA, WO 7/109, pp. 347–9.
52. 'Weir to McGrigor', 17 November 1812, TNA, WO 7/109, p. 375.
53. 'McGrigor to Wellington', 30 December 1812, WL, RAMC 799/6, p. 191–2.
54. Blanco, *Wellington's Surgeon General*, p. 139

55. Peterkin et al., *Commissioned Officers*, pp. 112, 137.
56. 'McGrigor to Gunning', 13 February 1814, WL, RAMC 799/6, (book II), p. 250.
57. 'McGrigor to AMB', 12 January 1813, WL, RAMC 799/6, pp. 202–3.
58. 'McGrigor to AMB', 21 February 1813, WL, RAMC 799/6, pp. 231.
59. 'McGrigor to Forbes', 19 May 1814, WL, RAMC 799/6, p. 363. See also the letters following to other senior medical officers.
60. These methods were not dissimilar to those which achieved prominence in the naval medical service around this time, and which have been discussed as being particularly well adapted to military enforcement by Lawrence, 'Disciplining Diseases'.
61. See for example, 'McGrigor to Wellington', 19 January 1814, WL, RAMC 799/8, pp. 153–4, regarding necessary modifications of the moveable hospitals.
62. See WL, RAMC 799/7, throughout.
63. McGrigor, 'Sketch of the Medical History', pp. 381–477.
64. 'McGrigor to Reed', 22 May 1812, WL, RAMC 799/6, p. 30.
65. McGrigor, 'Sketch of the Medical History', p. 408–9.
66. Ibid., p. 427.
67. Ibid., p. 428.
68. Ibid., p. 438.
69. 'McGrigor to Military Secretary', 3 November 1812, WL, RAMC 799/6, p. 144.
70. 'McGrigor to AMB', 22 November 1812, WL, RAMC 799/6, pp. 155–6.
71. 'Instructions for the Regulation of Military Hospitals and the Sick with Divisions of the Army in the Peninsula', Lisbon, 1813, WL, RAMC 149, p. 3
72. Ibid., p. 26.
73. Ibid., p. 77.
74. WL, RAMC 149, p. 47.
75. 'McGrigor to DI Higgins', 28 January 1814, WL, RAMC 799/6 (book II), p. 229.
76. Cook, 'Practical Medicine'.
77. 'Reed to McGrigor', 15 December 1812, TNA, WO 7/109, p. 386; see also: 'Weir and Kennedy to Grant', 6 October 1810, TNA, WO 7/107, p. 40; 'Reed to Grant', 6 December 1810, TNA, WO 7/107, p. 128; 'Reed to Grant', 6 November 1812, TNA, WO 7/108, p. 145.
78. McGrigor, 'Sketch of the Medical History', p. 418.
79. Ibid., pp. 449–59.
80. Ibid., p. 459.
81. 'Dent to his Cousin', 2 June 1814, WL, RAMC 536, Dent Letters, f. 31.
82. Gibney, *Eighty Years Ago*, p. 156
83. On issues of gender and types of medical practice, particularly the distinction between 'feminized' physic, and 'masculine' military surgeons, see M. Pelling, 'Compromised by Gender: The Role of the Male Medical Practitioners in Early Modern England', in H. Marland and M. Pelling (eds), *The Task of Healing, Medicine, Religion and Gender in England and the Netherlands, 1450–1800* (Rotterdam: Erasmus, 1996), pp. 101–33.
84. Gibney, *Eighty Years Ago*, p. 120.
85. Sherer, *Recollections*, p. 75.
86. Rosner, *The Most Beautiful Man*, p. 79.
87. A. Halliday, *Memoir of the Campaign of 1815* (Paris, 1816); Neale, *The Spanish Campaign of 1808*; Neale, *Letters*.
88. Halliday, *Observations*.

89. C. Boutflower, *The Journal of an Army Surgeon during the Peninsular War* (Staplehurst: Spellmount, 1997).
90. Commonplace book and travel diary of Thomas Thomson 1799–1852, WL, MS 4781.
91. Broughton, *Letters from Portugal, Spain and France*.
92. P. Hayward (ed.), *Surgeon Henry's Trifles, Events of a Military Life* (London: Chatto & Windus, 1970).
93. J. Vansittart (ed.), *Surgeon James's Journal 1815* (London: Cassell, 1964).
94. For a discussion of the picturesque and its adoption by the upper classes in this period see, L. Colley, *Britons, Forging the Nation 1707–1837*, 3rd edn (London: Yale University Press, 2005), pp. 172–4: 'one needed to have acquired a fashionable, aesthetic education: a knowledge of Edmund Burke's theory of the sublime, a properly developed understanding of the picturesque'. The ability to demonstrate these qualities in the description of a vista or landscape became 'a way of proclaiming who one was'.

6 Beyond the Wars

1. Ackroyd et al., *Advancing with the Army*, p. 220–1.
2. Ibid., p. 253.
3. B. Welsh, *A Practical Treatise on the Efficacy of Blood-Letting in the Epidemic Fever* (Edinburgh: Bell & Bradfute, 1819).
4. See Harrison, *Medicine in an Age of Commerce and Empire*, part 3, ch. 1.
5. Niebyl, 'The English Bloodletting Revolution', pp. 464–83.
6. Welsh, *A Practical Treatise*, p. 141.
7. Ackroyd et al., *Advancing with the Army*, p. 254.
8. W. Fergusson, 'A Letter to the Managers of the Royal Infirmary Edinburgh', Edinburgh, 1818, WL, RAMC 474/61, pp. 14–16.
9. See Blanco, *Wellington's Surgeon General*, ch. 9: 'McGrigor's Post-Waterloo reforms', for a detailed account of these innovations.
10. 'Public Health and Mortality', *Quarterly Review*, 66 (1840), pp. 115–55, on p. 116.
11. 'McGrigor to Thomson', 7 October 1815, GSC, MS Cullen, f. 886.
12. 'McGrigor to Thomson', 18 October 1815, GSC, MS Cullen, f. 887.
13. McGrigor, 'Sketch of the Medical History', p. 463.
14. Ibid., p. 464.
15. 'McGrigor to Thomson', 30 October 1815, GSC, MS Cullen, f. 884; 'McGrigor to Thomson', 2 October 1815, GSC, MS Cullen, f. 885.
16. 'McGrigor to Thomson', 9 February 1818, GSC, MS Cullen, f. 912.
17. Thomson provides an interesting study of a practitioner who grasped the potential of 'militarized' medicine prior to his even serving with the army, see: Jacyna, *Philosophic Whigs*.
18. 'McGrigor to Thomson', 22 July 1817, GSC, MS Cullen, f. 905; 'McGrigor to Thomson', 31 August 1814, GSC, MS Cullen, f. 906; 'McGrigor to Thomson', 19 September 1817, GSC, MS Cullen, f. 909; 'McGrigor to Thomson', 13 October 1817, GSC, MS Cullen f. 910; 'McGrigor to Thomson', 7 March 1818, GSC, MS Cullen, f. 913. Not that McGrigor also made the claim in these letters to have pursued the same treatment himself in India twenty years prior to the Peninsular War. For a report of trials being conducted by other medical practitioners see: 'G. Barclay to Thomson', 12 January 1818, GSC, MS Cullen, f. 971.
19. 'Circular on Syphilis', 2 April 1819, WL, MS Ballingall, 6905/7.

20. Copies of reports of Sir William Burnett 1822, Royal Naval Museum Library, Portsmouth, Burnett Papers, MS 242/1, pp. 64–6.
21. T. Rose, 'Observations on the Treatment of Syphilis, with an Account of Several Cases of that Disease in which a Cure was Effected Without the Use of Mercury', *Medico-Chirurgical Transactions*, 8 (1817), pp. 347–424; G. Guthrie, 'Observations on the Treatment of the Venereal Disease, Without Mercury' (London, 1817), annexed to H. Desruelles, *Memoir on the Treatment of Venereal Diseases Without Mercury, Employed at the Military Hospital of the Val-de-Grace* (Philadelphia: Carey & Lea, 1830); J. Thomson, 'Observations on the Treatment of Syphilis Without Mercury', *EMSJ*, 14 (1818), pp. 84–91.
22. '"Upon the Treatment of Syphilis without Mercury, with reference to the experiments lately made in Great Britain" by Dr Ferdinand William Becker, of Berlin. Translated from a paper in the Archiv. fur Mediziniche Erfarhung &c, Von Horn &c., for Jan and Feb. 1826', *London Medical Repository and Review*, 3 (1826), pp. 532–6, on p. 533.
23. Rose, 'Observations on the Treatment of Syphilis', pp. 361–2.
24. Ibid., p. 422.
25. J. Sainty, *The Origin of the Office of Chairman of Committees in the House of Lords* (House of Lords Record Office, 1974), p. 1, online at http://www.Parliament.uk/documents/upload/chairmn.pdf [accessed 7 July 2007].
26. The details of those inquiries can be found in: *Commons Journals*, 51, pp. 450, 512–17: 'Petition of Matthew Baillie physician and Everard Home, Esq, surgeon', 29 February 1796 and 16 March 1796; and in the following committee reports presented to Parliament: *CCR* (1801–2), 2:75, pp. 267–318: 'Report from the committee on Dr. Jenner's petition, respecting his discovery of vaccine Inoculation', 6 May 1802; *CCR* (1801–2), 2:114, pp. 381–499: 'Report from the committee on Dr. C. Smyth's petition, respecting his discovery of nitrous fumigation', 10 June 1802; *CCR* (1818), 7:285, pp. 59–71: 'Report from the select committee on the contagious fever in Ireland', 8 May 1818; *CCR* (1818), 7:332, pp. 1–52: 'Report from the select committee on contagious fever in London', 20 May 1818; *CCR* (1819), 2:449), pp. 537–638: 'Report from the select committee appointed to consider the validity of the doctrine of contagion in the plague'; *CCR* (1821), 4:732, pp. 335–40: 'Report from the select committee on the ophthalmic hospital', 3 July 1821; *CCR* (1824), 6:417, pp. 165–287: 'Second report from the select committee appointed to consider the means of improving and maintaining the foreign trade of the country', 14 June 1824. These are not the only select committees to have investigated matters related to medical questions, however they are the only ones which have any military focus or which consider a medical controversy.
27. The majority of these men have already appeared in preceding chapters and their connection with military medicine need not be reiterated. Robert Keate was the nephew of Thomas Keate and had been apprenticed to his uncle in 1792. He was appointed staff surgeon in the army in 1798 and rose to the rank of inspector-general of hospitals. He retired in 1810. See Bettany, 'Keate, Robert (1777–1857)', rev. Christian Kerslake, *ODNB*. Dr Joseph Marshall was physician extraordinary to the King of Naples and gave extensive testimony about, *inter alia*, the inoculation of soldiers and sailors in Gibraltar, Minorca, Malta and Sicily.
28. The best account of the inquiry is R. B. Fisher, *Edward Jenner, 1749–1823* (London: Andre Deutsch, 1991), which in ch. 6 contains a good review of the lead up to, and proceedings for, the presentation of the petition to Parliament as well as the workings of the select committee.

29. 'Report from the committee on Dr. Jenner's petition, respecting his discovery of vaccine Inoculation', p. 18.
30. Ibid., p. 14.
31. Dr Woodville, physician to the small pox hospital, Mr John Griffiths, surgeon to St Georges hospital, and Dr Nelson, physician to the vaccine pock Institution, all gave evidence of large numbers of inoculations within their establishments: 7,500; 1,500; and 700, respectively.
32. 'Manpower economy' arguments were also, at this time, being used more frequently by military practitioners in their writings; see for example the works of Gilbert Blane, James Johnson, Robert Robertson and Thomas Trotter.
33. G. Stronach, 'Smyth, James Carmichael (1742–1821)', rev. J. Loudon, *ODNB* http://www.oxforddnb.com/view/article/25950 [accessed 8 April 2008].
34. 'Report from the committee on Dr. C. Smyth's petition, respecting his discovery of nitrous fumigation', appendix no. 1.
35. Ibid., pp. 24–5; see also J. C. Smyth, *The Effect of the Nitrous Vapour, in Preventing and Destroying Contagion; Ascertained from a Variety of Trials, Made Chiefly by Surgeons of His Majesty's Navy, in Prisons, Hospitals, and on Board of Ships: With an Introduction Respecting the Nature of Contagion, which gives Rise to the Jail or Hospital Fever; And the Various Methods Formerly Employed to Prevent or Destroy This* (London: J. Johnson, 1799), p. 59.
36. For his account of these trials see J. C. Smyth, *An Account of the Experiment Made at the Desire of the Lords Commissioners of the Admiralty on Board the Union Hospital Ship to Determine the Effect of the Nitrous Acid in Destroying Contagion and the Safety with which it may be Employed, in a Letter Addressed to the Rt. Honorable Lord Spencer, &c., &c., &c.* (London: J. Johnson, 1796).
37. *Commons Journals*, 57, p. 173.
38. 'Report from the committee on Dr. C. Smyth's petition, respecting his discovery of nitrous fumigation', p. 4.
39. Ibid., pp. 4–5.
40. Ibid., p. 8.
41. Ibid., p. 41.
42. Ibid., pp. 45–9. Although the author of these letters is recorded as 'Mr. McGregor' his post as surgeon of the 88th Regiment at this time makes it clear the author is James McGrigor.
43. Ibid., p. 46.
44. Ibid., p. 47.
45. These inaccuracies should not have been fatal to his evidence and the committee's dismissal of Lind would appear to have more to do with his character and reliability as a disinterested man of his word, see Shapin, *A Social History of Truth* for the importance of such qualities in the preceding century.
46. 'Report from the committee on Dr. C. Smyth's petition, respecting his discovery of nitrous fumigation', p. 69.
47. Ibid., p. 73.
48. For a discussion of the rise of statistical record keeping and its use in medicine during this period see, Tröhler, '*To Improve the Evidence of Medicine*'.
49. 'Report from the committee on Dr. C. Smyth's petition, respecting his discovery of nitrous fumigation', p. 81.
50. Harrison, *Medicine in an Age of Commerce*.

51. 'Report from the committee on Dr. C. Smyth's petition, respecting his discovery of nitrous fumigation', p. 80.
52. Ibid., pp. 80–2.
53. Ibid., p. 7.
54. *Commons Journals*, 57, p. 565.
55. Ibid., p. 650.
56. Loudon, *Medical Care and the General Practitioner*, esp. ch. 7.
57. Ibid., p. 66. Cantlie, *A History*, makes brief reference to the proposed exclusion and the feelings of military practitioners at pp. 435–6; Ackroyd et al., *Advancing with the Army*, state: 'Army and naval surgeons were not affected by the legislation, but it is not hard to see that McGrigor would have been anxious to demonstrate to the public that his officers deserved their exemption on the grounds of their exemplary education', p. 57.
58. 'Doctor Latham, President of the Royal College of Physicians to the Rt Hon. George Rose', 27 January 1814, Apothecaries Hall, MS 8211/1, Act of Parliament Committee Minutes 1814–34, p. 7.
59. 23 August 1815, Act of Parliament Committee Minutes 1814–34, Apothecaries Hall, MS 8211/1, p. 87.
60. Act of Parliament Committee Minutes 1814–34, Apothecaries Hall, MS 8211/1, pp. 90–1; Extract from the Minutes of the Court of Examiners, 19 January 1816, Apothecaries Hall, MS 8211/1, p. 98; 'Opinion of C. Warren', 19 January 1816, Apothecaries Hall, MS 8211/1, pp. 99–100; 'Letter to Mr Buckler', 28 March 1816, Apothecaries Hall, MS 8211/1, p. 104.
61. 'Letter from the AMB Office', 19 April 1816, Act of Parliament Committee Minutes 1814–34, Apothecaries Hall, MS 8211/1 , p. 105.
62. Act of Parliament Committee Minutes 1814–34, Apothecaries Hall, MS 8211/1, p. 106.
63. Ibid.
64. Ibid.
65. Autobiographical details in Maclean' s published works provide the following brief biography: Maclean was born in around 1765, and by 1788 had obtained the degrees of physician and surgeon. He commenced practice as the surgeon of the East Indiaman, the *William Pitt*. In the service of the East India Company he travelled to Bengal, Jamaica and the East Indies. He left the Company's service in India, and in 1796 worked in the Mariner's Ward of the Calcutta general hospital. At this time he was also proprietor of a newspaper. In July 1798, he was ordered to leave India by Wellesley because of his criticism of a magistrate. After a year-long cruise he arrived in England and almost at once departed for Germany where he remained throughout most of 1800 and 1801 seeking opportunities for the study of epidemic diseases. In 1801 he moved to Paris and was there during Napoleon's detention of the English in France in 1802. On proving he had not been in England for ten years, he was permitted to leave France. In 1804, he applied for a position with the hospital staff of the British Army and served in York Hospital Chelsea, Chelmsford, Gosport and Cork until 1805. He left the service but was listed in the *Gazette* as 'superseded for being absent without leave' and in the *Hue and Cry* as a 'Deserter'. In 1810 he began lecturing on the 'Diseases of Hot Climates' under the sanction of the East India Company and in 1815 travelled to the Levant to 'investigate the plague'. From his return that year he agitated strenuously for reform to the quarantine laws, participating in both the 1819 and 1824 parliamentary inquiries. In 1821 he was commissioned by the Spanish government to investigate the fever in Barcelona and

was successful in persuading the Cortes to overturn their sanitary laws. Publications and letters to periodicals from Maclean cease after 1826; see also M. Harrison, 'Maclean, Charles (fl. 1788–1824)', *ODNB*, online at http://www.oxforddnb.com/view/article/17649 [accessed 24 May 2006].

66. For a detailed description of Maclean's medical philosophy see C. Kelly, '"Not from the College, but through the Public and the Legislature": Charles Maclean and the Relocation of Medical Debate in the Early 19th Century', *Bulletin of the History of Medicine*, 82 (2008), pp. 545–69; and Harrison, *Medicine in an Age of Commerce*.

67. On Maclean's strategy see Kelly, '"Not from the College"'.

68. See Maclean's account of his correspondence with these persons and companies detailed throughout C. Maclean, *Specimens of Systematic Misrule* (London: H. Hay, 1820); also BL, Add. 59265, Dropmore Papers, ff. 92–188.

69. C. Maclean, *Results of an Investigation Regarding Epidemic and Pestilential Diseases Including Researches in the Levant, Concerning the Plague*, 2 vols (London: Underwood, 1817 and 1818).

70. BL, Add. 59265, Dropmore Papers, f. 175.

71. *Commons Journals*, 74, p. 122: The committee ordered comprised: Sir John Jackson, Mr Bennet, Mr Boswell, Mr Fowell Buxton, Mr Henry Clive, Mr Cust, Mr Dawson, Mr Fazakerley, Mr Fleming, Mr Davies Gilbert, Mr Sandford Graham, Mr Hudson Gurney, Mr Heygate, Mr Legh, Mr Macqueen, Sir Charles Monck, Mr Morritt, Dr. Phillimore, Mr Frederick Robinson, Mr Wallace and Mr Wilberforce.

72. Jackson was born in Jamaica in 1763, the son of a surgeon. He entered Parliament in 1806 as the member for Dover. In April 1807, he became a director of the East India Company. For further details see his biographical entry in R. G. Thorne (ed.), *The History of Parliament: House of Commons 1790–1820* (London: Secker & Warburg for the History of Parliament Trust, 1986).

73. *Hansard*, 40 (1819), pp. 1133–34.

74. 'Report from the Select Committee … Doctrine of Contagion', p. 97.

75. 'Second Report from the select committee'.

76. *Hansard*, n.s., 12 (1825), pp. 993–6.

77. Ibid., p. 1315.

78. G. Blane, *Elements of Medical Logick* (London: Underwood, 1819), p. 181.

79. Ibid., p. 182.

80. 'Critical Analysis', *EMSJ*, 24 (1825), p. 100.

81. C. Maclean, 'On the Monopoly of the College of Physicians', *Medical Observer*, 1 (1807), pp. 300–24; 'Dr. Maclean's Second Letter on the Monopoly of the College of Physicians', *Medical Observer*, (January 1808), pp. 345–87; 'Dr. Maclean's Third Letter on the Monopoly of the College of Physicians', *Medical Observer*, 2 (February 1808), pp. 52–70.

82. 'Report from the select committee … doctrine of contagion', p. 100.

83. 'Second report from the select committee', pp. 237–8. Although Granville had served with the Royal Navy during the Wars, his membership of a noble Italian family, classical education, association with elite London society and successful civilian practice in obstetrics after 1812 set him within the 'establishment'. He was a licentiate of the Royal College of Physicians, and a Fellow of the Royal Society. See W. Howell, 'Augustus Bozzi Granville – Journeyman Physician', *Canadian Medical Association Journal*, 25 (1931), pp. 719–25.

84. Blane, *Elements of Medical Logick*, pp. 92, 96. Blane was a licentiate of the Royal College of Physicians, had a very successful civilian practice in addition to his appointments with the Navy and held a series of Royal appointments. He was a close associate of Sir Lucas Pepys (see Chapter 2). See J. Wallace, 'Blane, Sir Gilbert, first baronet (1749–1834)', *ODNB*, online at http://www.oxforddnb.com/view/article/2621 [accessed 30 September 2008].

85. 'Report from the select committee ... doctrine of contagion', p. 29.

86. 'Plague a Contagious Disease', *Quarterly Review*, 33 (1825), p. 239; 'Review of Tully and Hancock', *Medico-Chirurgical Review*, 2 (1821), p. 570.

87. 'We are glad to see a bill in progress for the revision of the Quarantine Laws', *The Times Digital Archive*, 2 April 1825.

88. *Hansard*, n.s., 13 (1825), p. 603.

89. *Hansard*, n.s., 12 (1825), p. 1326.

90. For an overview of his career see W. Courtney, 'Adams, Sir William (1783–1827)', rev. J. Tiffany, *ODNB*, online at http://www.oxforddnb.com/view/article/23200 [accessed 18 April 2006].

91. W. Adams, *A Letter to the Right Honourable and Honourable the Directors of Greenwich Hospital, Containing an Exposure of the Measures Resorted to, by the Medical Officers of the London Eye Infirmary, for the Purpose of Retarding the Adoption, and Execution of Plans for the Extermination of the Egyptian Ophthalmia from the Army, and from the Kingdom, Submitted for the Approval of Government* (London: Baldwin Cradock & Joy, 1817).

92. *Official Papers Relating to Operations Performed by Order of the Directors of the Royal Hospital for Seamen, at Greenwich, on Several of the Pensioners Belonging thereto, for the Purpose of Ascertaining the General Efficacy of the New Modes of Treatment Practised by Sir William Adams, for the Cure of the Various Species of Cataract, and the Egyptian Ophthalmia, Published by Order of the Directors* (London: Manufactory for Employment of Deaf & Dumb, 1814).

93. Anon., *Facts and Documents Relating to the Establishment of the Ophthalmic Hospital* (London: L. Harrison, 1821).

94. Ibid.

95. Ibid., p. 3.

96. *Official Papers Relating to Operations Performed*, p. iv.

97. Ibid., p. 8.

98. Ibid., p. iv.

99. Anon., *Facts and Documents*, p. 4.

100. Ibid., p. 4.

101. Ibid., p. 8; Adams's claims regarding the hostility of army medical practitioners are repeated in private letters to Lord Palmerston, see 'Adams to Palmerson', 5 December 1816, BL, Add. 48432, Palmerston Papers, ff. 129–32; Memoranda [unattributed], BL, Add. 48436, Palmerston Papers, f. 162; and the 2nd Earl of Liverpool, see 'Adams to Liverpool', 21 June 1817, BL, Add. 38267, Liverpool Papers, f. 157; and 'Adams to Liverpool', 24 June 1817, BL, Add. 38267, Liverpool Papers, ff. 188–95.

102. J. Vetch, *Observations Relative to the Treatment by Sir William Adams, of the Ophthalmic Cases of the Army* (London: J. Davy for J. Callow, 1818).

103. 'Sir W. Adams and Dr. Vetch on Ophthalmia', *EMSJ*, 14 (1818), pp. 223–36; The involvement of political patrons on Adams's behalf is alluded to by McGrigor in a letter written in 1817: 'Lord Melville is an ally of Adams', see 'McGrigor to Irwin', 18 September 1817, GSC, MS Cullen, f. 969.

104. Courtney, 'Adams , Sir William'

105. Vetch, *Observations*, p. 5–6.
106. Ibid., p. 8.
107. Ibid., p. 19. Vetch used graduated application of caustic substances.
108. Ibid., p. 21.
109. W. Adams, *A Reply by Sir William Adams to a Pamphlet Recently Published by Dr. Vetch, upon the Subject of the Egyptian Ophthalmia and to Other Productions of a Similar Character* (London: J. Callow, 1818).
110. For a statement of the bleeding treatment see: J. Vetch, *A Practical Treatise on the Diseases of the Eye* (London: G. & W. B. Whittaker, 1820).
111. *Hansard*, 10 May 1819, p. 316.
112. Ibid., p. 317.
113. Ibid., p. 318.
114. Ibid., p. 323.
115. Ibid., p. 330.
116. J. Vetch, *A Letter to the Rt. Hon. Lord Viscount Palmerston, Secretary at War, &c. &c. on the Subject of the Ophthalmic Institution for the Cure of Chelsea Pensioners*, 2nd edn (London, 1819).
117. Ibid., p. 22.
118. Ibid., p. 3.
119. Ibid., p. 25.
120. Ibid., pp. 26–7.
121. *The Times Digital Archive*, 7 March 1821, p. 2.
122. 'Report from the select committee on the ophthalmic hospital'.
123. *The Times Digital Archive*, 11 July 1821, p. 2; 25 July 1822, p. 2.
124. Chelsea Hospital, *Report to HRH the Commander-in-Chief upon the Subject of the Out Pensioners of Chelsea Hospital, that have been Under Treatment for Diseases of the Eyes: Also, the Reports Made by the Medical Officers of Chelsea Hospital upon the Cases of those Patients* (London: J. Reed, 1819).
125. *The Times Digital Archive*, 11 July 1821, p. 2. Unfortunately, I have been unable to discover any official record of the proceedings before this select committee.
126. 'Pamphlets on the Ophthalmic Question', *EMSJ*, 17 (1821), pp. 608–19.
127. Ibid., p. 619.
128. The Committee ordered on 10 May 1821 included: Lord Viscount Palmerston, Mr Chancellor of the Exchequer Nicholas Vannisttart, Sir Thomas Acland, Mr George Banks, Mr Joseph Foster Barham, Mr Grey Bennett, Mr George Dawson, Lord Viscount Ebrington, Sir Ronald Ferguson, Mr Grant, Mr Holmes, Mr Hutchinson, Sir Charles Long, Sir James Mackintosh, Mr Tremayne and Mr Wilmot, *Commons Journals*, 76, p. 325; Sir Thomas Pechell, joined on 10 May 1821, *Commons Journals*, 76, p. 330; Sir Lowry Cole, Sir Henry Hardinge and Mr Wood joined on 14 May 1821, *Commons Journals*, 76, p. 341; Mr O'Grady and Mr Macqueen joined on 15 May 1821, *Commons Journals*, 76, p. 345.
129. S. E. Finer, 'The Transmission of Benthamite Ideas 1820–50', in G. Sutherland (ed.), *Studies in the Growth of Nineteenth-Century Government* (London: Routledge and Kegan Paul, 1972), pp. 11–32.
130. Specifically, Banks's influence as the central point in a 'Republic of Letters', and as the acknowledged advisor to government on scientific matters. On these aspects of Banks's career see J. Gascoigne, *Science in the Service of Empire, Joseph Banks, the British State and the uses of Science in the Age of Revolutions* (Cambridge: Cambridge University Press, 1998).

WORKS CITED

Manuscript and Archival Sources

Apothecaries Hall, London.

MS 8211/1, Act of Parliament Committee Minutes 1814–34.

British Library, London.

Add. 59265, Dropmore Papers.

Add. 38267, Liverpool Papers.

Add. 48436, Palmerston Papers.

The National Archives, London.

WO 1, Secretary at war, secretary of state for war and commander-in-chief, in-letters and miscellaneous papers.

WO 4, Secretary at war, out-letters.

WO 7, War Office and predecessors: various departmental out-letters.

WO 40, War Office: secretary at war, in-letters and reports.

WO 123, Ministry of Defence and predecessors: Army circulars, memoranda, orders and regulations.

WO 134, War Office: General Sir W. Marmaduke Peacocke, Commander at Lisbon: papers.

The Wellcome Library, London.

RAMC 149, 'Instructions for the regulation of military hospitals and the sick with divisions of the army in the Peninsula ...'

RAMC 208, Fergusson Papers.

RAMC 210, Fergusson Papers.

RAMC 211, Fergusson Papers.

RAMC 212, Fergusson Papers.

RAMC 474/61, Parkes Pamphlet Collection.

RAMC 536, Dent Letters.

RAMC 715/5, 'James Dickson, M.A. 1769–1795, Army Surgeon'.

RAMC 799, McGrigor Papers.

RAMC 830, Murray Papers.

MS 1529, Catherwood Papers.

MS 4781, Thomson Papers.

University of Glasgow Library, Special Collections.

MS Cullen 880–974, Thompson Papers.

British Newspapers and Periodicals

Colburn's United Service Magazine and Naval and Military Journal.

Edinburgh Medical and Surgical Journal.

Lancet.

London Medical and Surgical Spectator.

Medical and Physical Journal.

Medical Observer.

Medico-Chirurgical Review.

Medico-Chirurgical Transactions.

Quarterly Review.

Times.

Transactions of a Society for the Improvement of Medical and Chirurgical Knowledge.

Parliamentary Papers

Cobbett's Parliamentary Debates.

General Indexes to the *Commons Journals* for the years 1697–1800.

Commons Journals.

Commons Committee Reports.

Hansard.

House of Commons Sessional Papers.

Primary Sources

Adams, W., *A Letter to the Right Honourable and Honourable the Directors of Greenwich Hospital, Containing an Exposure of the Measures Resorted to, by the Medical Officers of the London Eye Infirmary, for the Purpose of Retarding the Adoption, and Execution of Plans for the Extermination of the Egyptian Ophthalmia from the Army, and from the Kingdom, Submitted for the Approval of Government* (London: Baldwin Cradock & Joy, 1817).

—, *A Reply by Sir William Adams to a Pamphlet Recently Published by Dr. Vetch, upon the Subject of the Egyptian Ophthalmia and to Other Productions of a Similar Character* (London: J. Callow, 1818).

Alpinus, P., *La médicine des Egyptiens 1581–1584 traduite du latin, et anotée par R. de Fenol* (Cairo: Institut francais d'archaeologie orientale du Caire, 1980).

Anon., 'Of the Practice of Medicine in Great Britain, as Conducted by Physicians, Surgeons, Apothecaries, &c. &c.', *Medical Observer*, 1 (1806), p. 195.

—, *Memoirs Relative to Egypt, Written in that Country during the Campaigns of General Bonaparte, in the Years 1798 and 1799, by the Learned and Scientific Men who Accompanied the French Expedition* (London: T. Gillet for R. Phillips, 1800).

—, *Identities Ascertained or, An Illustration of Mr Ware's Opinion Respecting the Sameness of Infection in Venereal Gonorrhaea, and the Pphthalmia of Egypt: With an Examination of Affinity between Antient Leprosy and Lues* (London: J. & W. Smith, 1808).

—, *Facts and Documents Relating to the Establishment of the Ophthalmic Hospital* (London: L. Harrison, 1821).

—, 'Journal of a Soldier of the LXXI Regiment from 1806 to 1815', in *Constable's Miscellany of Original and Selected Publications in the Various Departments of Literature, Science and the Arts* (Edinburgh, 1828), vol. 27, p. 69.

Assalini, P., *Observations on the Disease Called the Plague, on the Dysentery, the Ophthalmy of Egypt, and on the Means of Prevention with some Remarks on the Yellow Fever of Cadiz, and the Description and Plan of an Hospital for the Reception of Patients Affected with Epidemic and Contagious Diseases. Translated from the French by Adam Neale of the University of Edinburgh, Member of the Royal College of Surgeons of that City, and Late Surgeon of the Shropshire Regiment of Militia* (New York: T. & J. Swords, 1806).

Bancroft, E., *A Letter to the Commissioners of Military Enquiry: Containing Animadversions on Some Parts of Their Fifth Report; And an Examination of the Principles on which the Medical Department of the Armies Ought to be Formed* (London: T. Cadell and W. Davies, 1808).

—, *An Exposure and Refutation of Various Misrepresentations Published by Dr McGrigor and Dr Jackson, in their Separate Letters to the Commissioners of Military Enquiry; Interspersed with Facts and Observations Concerning Military Hospitals and Medical Arrangements for Armies* (London: T. Cadell & W. Davies, 1808).

Bell, J., *Memorial Concerning the Present State of Military and Naval Surgery Addressed Several Years Ago to the Right Honorable Earl Spencer, First Lord of the Admiralty; And Now Submitted to the Public* (Edinburgh: Longman & Rees, 1800).

Blane, G., 'To the Editors of the Medical and Physical Journal', *Medical and Physical Journal*, 6 (1801), p. 357.

—, 'Statements of the Comparative Health of the British Navy, from the Year 1779 to the Year 1814, with Proposals for its Farther Improvement', *Medico-Chirurgical Transactions*, 6 (1815), pp. 490–573.

—, *Elements of Medical Logick* (London: Underwood, 1819).

Borland, J., 'Copy of a Letter from Dr. Borland, to the Inspector Generals of Army Hospitals; dated 20th June 1808', in *Papers Relating to the Army Medical Board* (Ordered, by the House of Commons, to be printed, 4 May 1810, London, 1810).

Boutflower, C., *The Journal of an Army Surgeon during the Peninsular War* (Staplehurst: Spellmount, 1997).

Broughton, S., *Letters from Portugal, Spain and France* (1815; Stroud: Nonsuch, 2005).

Bruant, 'Account of the Prevailing Ophthalmia of Egypt, by Citizen Bruant, Physician in Ordinary to the Army, Head Quarters at Cairo, 15th Fructidor, 6th Year', in Anon., *Memoirs Relative to Egypt*, pp. 110–18.

Bruce, N., 'Remarks on the Dracunculus, or Guinea Worm, as it Appeared in the Peninsula of India', *EMSJ*, 2 (1806), pp. 145–50.

Chelsea Hospital, *Report to HRH the Commander-in-Chief upon the Subject of the Out Pensioners of Chelsea Hospital, that have been Under Treatment for Diseases of the Eyes: Also, the Reports Made by the Medical Officers of Chelsea Hospital upon the Cases of those Patients* (London: J. Reed, 1819).

Costello, E., *The Adventures of a Soldier; Or Memoirs of Edward Costello K.S.F., Formerly a Non-Commissioned Officer in the Rifle Brigade, and Late Captain in the British Legion* (London: Henry Colburn, 1841).

Desgenettes, R., 'Circular Letter, from Citizen Desgenettes, to the Medical Men of the Army of the East, Relative to a Plan for Drawing up a Physico-Medical Topography of Egypt', in Anon., *Memoirs Relative to Egypt*, p. 67.

—, *Histoire médicale de l'armee d'orient, par le medecin en chief R. Desgenettes* (Paris: Croullebois & Bossange, 1802).

Dewar, H., *Dissertatio medica inauguralis, de ophthalmia Ægypti : quam ... pro gradu doctoris ...* (Edinburgh: Creech, 1804).

—, *Observations on Diarrhoea and Dysentery, Particularly as these Diseases Appeared in the British Campaign of Egypt in 1801* (London: John Murray, 1805).

Edmonston, A., *A Treatise on the Varieties and Consequences of Ophthalmia with a Preliminary Inquiry into its Contagious Nature* (Edinburgh: W. Blackwood, 1806).

Farrell, C., *Observations on Ophthalmia and its Consequences* (London: John Murray, 1811).

Fergusson, J. (ed.), *William Fergusson, Notes and Recollections of a Professional Life* (London: Longman, Brown, Green & Longmans, 1846).

'Fifth Report of the Commissioners of Military Enquiry', *HCSP*, 5 (1808), pp. 4–7.

'Further Observations on the Egyptian Ophthalmia, as it Affected the 2nd Battalion of the 52nd Regiment. In a Letter from George Peach, Esq. Surgeon to the 2nd Battalion 52nd Regiment, to James M'Gregor, M.D. Fellow of the Royal College of Physicians, Edinburgh, and Deputy Inspector-General of Hospitals, Portsmouth', *EMSJ*, 3 (1807), pp. 395–400.

Gibney, R. (ed.), *Eighty Years Ago, or the Recollections of an Old Army Doctor, His Adventures on the Field of Quatre Bras and Waterloo and during the Occupation of Paris in 1815, by the Late Dr. Gibney of Cheltenham* (London: Bellairs & Company, 1896).

Gurwood, J. (ed.), *The General Orders of Field Marshal the Duke of Wellington K. D. &c. &c .&c. in Portugal, Spain, and France, from 1809 to 1814; and the Low Countries and France, 1815* (London: Clowes & Sons, 1832).

—, *The Dispatches of Field Marshal the Duke of Wellington: During his Various Campaigns in India, Denmark, Portugal, Spain, the Low Countries, and France, from 1799 to 1818*, 13 vols (London: John Murray, 1838), vol. 7.

Guthrie, G., 'Observations on the Treatment of the Venereal Disease, Without Mercury' (London, 1817), annexed to H. Desruelles, *Memoir on the Treatment of Venereal Diseases Without Mercury, Employed at the Military Hospital of the Val-de-Grace* (Philadelphia: Carey & Lea, 1830).

Hall, S., 'Some Account of a Recent French Publication, Respecting the Pestilential and Malignant Fevers of the Levant', *Medical and Physical Journal*, 8 (1802), pp. 449–53

Halliday, A., *Observations on the Present State of the Portuguese Army, As Organised by Lieutenant-General Sir William Carr Beresford, K. B. Field Marshall and Commander in Chief of that Army. With an Account of the Different Military Establishments and Laws of Portugal, and a Sketch of the Campaigns of the Last and Present Year, during which the Portuguese Army was Brought into the Field Against the Enemy, for the First Time as a Regular Force* (London: John Murray, 1811).

—, *Memoir of the Campaign of 1815* (Paris, 1816).

Hamilton, R., *The Duties of a Regimental Surgeon Considered with Observations on his General Qualifications; And Hints Relative to a More Respectable Practice, and Better Regulation of that Department*, 2nd edn (London: printed by George Woodfall, for T. N. Longman; J. Johnson; and P. Foster, Ipswich, 1794).

Hayward, P. (ed.), *Surgeon Henry's Trifles, Events of a Military Life* (London: Chatto & Windus, 1970).

Hibbert, C. (ed.), *The Recollections of Rifleman Harris as told to Henry Curling* (London: Century, 1985).

—, *Corunna* (Moreton-In-Marsh: Windrush, 1996).

Hooper, R., 'Account of the Diseases of the Sick Landed at Plymouth from Corunna', *EMSJ*, 5 (1809), pp. 398–420.

Jackson, R., *A Treatise on the Fevers of Jamaica, with some Observations on the Intermitting Fever of America, and an Appendix Containing some Hints on the Means of Preserving the Health of Soldiers in Hot Climates* (London: John Murray, 1791).

—, *An Outline of the History and Cure of Fever, Endemic and Contagious; More Expressly the Contagious Fever of Jails, Ships, and Hospitals; The Concentrated Endemic, Vulgarly the Yellow Fever of the West Indies. To which is Added, an Explanation of the Principles of Military Discipline and Economy; With a Scheme of Medical Arrangement for Armies* (Edinburgh: Printed for Mundell & Son, 1798).

—, *Remarks on the Constitution of the Medical Department of the British Army: With a Detail of Hospital Management, and an Appendix, Attempting to Explain the Action of Causes in Producing Fever, and the Operation of Remedies in Effecting Cure* (London: T. Cadell and W. Davies, 1803).

—, *A Systematic View of the Formation, Discipline, and Economy of Armies* (London: John Stockdale, 1804).

—, *A System of Arrangement and Discipline, for the Medical Department of Armies* (London: John Murray, 1805).

—, *A Letter to the Commissioners of Military Enquiry; Explaining the True Constitution of a Medical Staff, the Best Form of Economy for Hospitals &c. With a Refutation of Errors and Misrepresentations Contained in a letter by Dr Bancroft Army Physician, dated 28 April 1808* (London: the author, 1808).

—, *A Letter to Mr Keate, Surgeon General to the Forces* (London: John Murray, 1808).

Keate, T., *Observations on the Fifth Report of the Commissioners of Military Enquiry and More Particularly on Those Parts of it which Relate to the Surgeon General* (London: J. Hatchard, 1808).

Larrey, D., *Memoirs of Military Surgery: And Campaigns of the French Armies, on the Rhine, in Corsica, Catalonia, Egypt, and Syria; At Boulogne, Ulm, and Austerlitz; in Saxony, Prussia, Poland, Spain, and Austria / from the French of D. J. Larrey ... by Richard Willmott Hall ... with Notes by the Translator* (Birmingham, AL: Classics of Surgery Library Division of Gryphon Editions, Ltd, 1985).

Lempriere, W., *Practical Observations on the Diseases of the Army in Jamaica, As they Occurred Between the Years 1792 and 1797*, 2 vols (London: T. N. Longman & O. Rees, 1799).

Lind, J., *An Essay on Diseases Incidental to Europeans in Hot Climates with the Method of Preventing Their Fatal Consequences* (London: T. Becket & P.A. de Hondt, 1768).

Maclean, C., 'On the Monopoly of the College of Physicians', *Medical Observer*, 1 (1807), pp. 300–24.

—, *An Analytical View of the Medical Department of the British Army* (London: J. J. Stockdale, 1810).

—, *Results of an Investigation Regarding Epidemic and Pestilential Diseases Including Researches in the Levant, Concerning the Plague*, 2 vols (London: Underwood, 1817 and 1818).

—, *Specimens of Systematic Misrule* (London: H. Hay, 1820).

McGrigor, J., *Medical Sketches of the Expedition from Egypt to India* (London: John Murray, 1804).

—, 'A Memoir on the State of Health of the 88th Regiment, and of the Corps Attached to it, from 1st June 1800 to the 31st May 1801, as Originally Presented to the Medical Board, Bombay', *EMSJ*, 1 (1805), pp. 266–89.

—, *A Letter to the Commissioners of Military Enquiry, In reply to Some Animadversions of Dr E. Nathaniel Bancroft on their Fifth Report* (London: John Murray, 1808).

—, 'Observations on the Fever which Appeared in the Army from Spain on their Return to this Country in January 1809', *EMSJ*, 6 (1810), pp. 19–32.

—, 'Sketch of the Medical History of the British Armies in the Peninsula of Spain and Portugal during the Late Campaigns', *Medico-Chirurgical Transactions*, 6 (1815), pp. 381–489.

McGrigor, M. (ed.), *Sir James McGrigor. The Scalpel and the Sword. The Autobiography of the Father of Army Medicine* (Dalkeith: Scottish Cultural Press, 2000).

McLean, H., *An Enquiry into the Nature, and Causes of the Great Mortality Among the Troops at St. Domingo: With Practical Remarks on the Fever of that Island* (London: Printed for T. Cadell, 1797).

Monro, D., *Observations on the Means of Preserving the Health of Soldiers*, 2nd edn, 2 vols (London: John Murray, 1780).

Neale, A., *Letters from Portugal and Spain; Comprising an Account of the Operations of the Armies under their Excellencies Sir Arthur Wellesley and Sir John Moore, from the Landing of the Troops in Mondego Bay to the Battle at Corunna* (London: T Gillet, 1809).

Nisbet, W., 'On the 5th Report of the Commissioners of Military Enquiry, on the Medical Department of the Army', *London Medical and Surgical Spectator*, 1 (1808), pp. 122–31 on p. 127.

'Observations on the Epidemic Ophthalmia, as it Affected the Troops in Hythe Barracks. In a Letter from George Peach, Esq. Surgeon of the 2d Battalion 52nd Foot, at Reading-Street Barracks, Kent, to James McGrigor, M.D. Deputy Inspector-General of Hospitals, Portsmouth', *EMSJ*, 3 (1807), pp. 52–5.

'Observations on the History and Treatment of an Epidemic Ophthalmia, which Appeared in the Fourth Battalion of the Royals, in Edinburgh Castle, during the Months of July and August 1807, By C.F. Forbes, Esq. Surgeon of the Royals', *EMSJ*, 3 (1807), pp. 430–4.

Official Papers Relating to Operations Performed by Order of the Directors of the Royal Hospital for Seamen, at Greenwich, on Several of the Pensioners Belonging thereto, for the Purpose of Ascertaining the General Efficacy of the New Modes of Treatment Practised by Sir William Adams, for the Cure of the Various Species of Cataract, and the Egyptian Ophthalmia, Published by Order of the Directors (London: Manufactory for Employment of Deaf & Dumb, 1814).

Power, G., *Attempt to Investigate the Cause of Egyptian Ophthalmia, with Observations on its Nature and Different Modes of Cure* (London: John Murray, 1803).

Pringle, J., *Observations on the Diseases of the Army*, 6th edn (London: Printed for A. Millar & T. Cadell, D. Wilson, T. Durham and T. Payne, 1768).

Proceedings and Report of a Special Medical Board Appointed by His Royal Highness the Commander in Chief, and the Secretary at War to Examine the State of the Hospital at the Military Depot in the Isle of Wight, &c. &c. &c. (London: L. B. Seeley, 1808).

'Remarks on the Difference between the Infectious Ophthalmia, and that Produced by the Artful Application of Irritating Substances to the Eyes. By John Vetch, M.D. Assistant Surgeon with Ophthalmia Detachments at Riding Street Barracks', *EMSJ*, 4 (1808), pp. 157–9.

Rose, T., 'Observations on the Treatment of Syphilis, with an Account of Several Cases of that Disease in which a Cure was Effected Without the Use of Mercury', *Medico-Chirurgical Transactions*, 8 (1817), pp. 347–424.

Russell, P., *A Treatise of the Plague Containing an Historical Journal and Medical Account of the Plague at Aleppo, in the years 1760, 1761 and 1762* (London: G. G. J. and J. Robinson, 1791).

Savaresi, A., 'Essai sur la topographie physique et médicale de Daimiette, suivi d'observations sur les maladies qui ont régné dans cette place, pendant le premiere semester de l'an VII, par le citoyen Savaresi, médecin ordinaire de l'armée', in Desgenettes, *Histoire médicale*, p. 86.

—, 'Description et traitement de l'optalmie d'Egypte, par le citoyen Savaresi, médecin ordinaire d'armée d'orient', in Desgenettes, *Histoire médicale*, p. 91.

Schaumann, A., *On the Road with Wellington, The Diary of a War Commissary in the Peninsular Campaigns*, ed. and trans. A. M. Ludovici (London: W. Heinemann, 1924).

Sherer, J., *Recollections of the Peninsula, by the Author of Sketches of India,* 2nd edn (London: Longman et al., 1824).

Sinnott, N., *Observations, Tending to Shew the Mismanagement of the Medical Department in the Army; With a View to Trace the Evils to their Source: And to Point out to Government the Necessity of Attending More to the Health of the Soldier in Time of War. To which is Annexed, a Representation of the System Adopted in the Hanoverian Service* (London: For J. Murray & S. Highley, 1796).

Smyth, J. C., *An Account of the Experiment Made at the Desire of the Lords Commissioners of the Admiralty on Board the Union Hospital Ship to Determine the Effect of the Nitrous Acid in Destroying Contagion and the Safety with which it may be Employed, in a Letter Addressed to the Rt. Honorable Lord Spencer, &c., &c., &c* (London: J. Johnson, 1796).

—, *The Effect of the Nitrous Vapour, in Preventing and Destroying Contagion; Ascertained from a Variety of Trials, Made Chiefly by Surgeons of His Majesty's Navy, in Prisons, Hospitals, and on Board of Ships: With an Introduction Respecting the Nature of Contagion, which gives Rise to the Jail or Hospital Fever; And the Various Methods Formerly Employed to Prevent or Destroy This* (London: J. Johnson, 1799).

Thomson, J., 'Observations on the Treatment of Syphilis Without Mercury', *EMSJ*, 14 (1818), pp. 84–91.

Vansittart J. (ed.), *Surgeon James's Journal 1815* (London: Cassell, 1964).

Verney, H. (ed.), *The Journals and Correspondence of General Sir Harry Calvert, Bart ... Comprising the Campaigns in Flanders and Holland in 1793–4* (London: Hurst & Blackett, 1853).

Vetch, J., *An Account of the Ophthalmia which has Appeared in England since the Return of the British Army from Egypt* (London, 1807).

—, *Observations Relative to the Treatment by Sir William Adams, of the Ophthalmic Cases of the Army* (London: J. Davy for J. Callow, 1818).

—, *A Letter to the Rt. Hon. Lord Viscount Palmerston, Secretary at War, &c. &c. on the Subject of the Ophthalmic Institution for the Cure of Chelsea Pensioners*, 2nd edn (London, 1819).

—, *A Practical Treatise on the Diseases of the Eye* (London: G. & W. B. Whittaker, 1820).

Ware, J., *Remarks on the Purulent Ophthalmy, which has Lately been Epidemical in this Country* (London: J. Mawman, 1808).

Welsh, B., *A Practical Treatise on the Efficacy of Blood-Letting in the Epidemic Fever* (Edinburgh: Bell & Bradfute, 1819).

Whyte, D., 'Mode of Managing Ocular Inflammations', *Medical and Physical Journal*, 7 (1802), pp. 209–16.

Wilson, R., *History of the British Expedition to Egypt; To which is Subjoined, A Sketch of the Present State of that Country and its Means of Defence. Illustrated with Maps, and a Portrait of Sir Ralph Abercromby*, 2nd edn (London: C. Roworth, 1803).

Wittman, W., *Travels in Turkey, Asia-Minor, Syria and Across the Desert into Egypt during the Years 1799, 1800, and 1801, in Company with the Turkish Army, and the British Military Mission. To which are Annexed, Observations on the Plague, and on the Diseases Prevalent in Turkey, and a Meteorological Journal* (London: T. Gillet, 1803).

Secondary Sources

Ackerknecht, E. H., *Medicine at the Paris Hospital, 1794–1848* (Baltimore, MD: Johns Hopkins Press, 1967).

—, 'Broussais, or A Forgotten Medical Revolution', *Bulletin of the History of Medicine*, 27 (1953), pp. 320–43.

Ackroyd, M., L. Brockliss, M. Moss, K. Retford and J. Stevenson, *Advancing with the Army, Medicine, the Professions, and Social Mobility in the British Isles, 1790–1850* (Oxford: Oxford University Press, 2006).

Bettany, G., 'Gunning, John (*d.* 1798)', rev. M. Bevan, in *ODNB*, online at http://www.oxforddnb.com/view/article/11747 [accessed 14 March 2008].

—, 'Keate, Thomas (1745–1821)', rev. M. Bevan, in *ODNB*, online at http://www.oxforddnb.com/view/article/15222 [accessed 14 March 2008].

Blanco, R. L., 'The Development of British Military Medicine, 1793–1814', *Military Affairs*, 38 (1974), pp. 4–10.

—, *Wellington's Surgeon General: Sir James Macgrigor* (Durham, NC: Duke University Press, 1974).

—, 'The Soldier's Friend – Sir Jeremiah Fitzpatrick, Inspector of Health for Land Forces', *Medical History*, 20 (1976), pp. 402–21.

Brett-James, A., 'The Walcheren Failure: Part One', *History Today*, 13 (1963), pp. 811–20.

—, 'The Walcheren Failure: Part Two' *History Today*, 14 (1964), pp. 60–8.

Brockliss, L., and C. Jones, *The Medical World of Early Modern France* (Oxford: Clarendon Press, 1997).

Brockliss, L., J. Cardwell and M. Moss, *Nelson's Surgeon, William Beatty, Naval Medicine, and the Battle of Trafalgar* (Oxford: Oxford University Press, 2005).

Bynum, W. F., 'Cullen and the Study of Fevers in Britain, 1760–1820', in W. F. Bynum and V. Nutton (eds), *Theories of Fever from Antiquity to the Enlightenment* (London: Wellcome Institute for the History of Medicine, 1981), pp. 135–47.

Bynum, W. F., and R. Porter (eds), *Brunonianism in Britain and Europe* (London: Wellcome Institute for the History of Medicine, 1988).

Cantlie, N., *A History of the Army Medical Department*, 2 vols (Edinburgh and London: Churchill Livingstone, 1974), vol. 1.

Chandler, D., 'The Egyptian Campaign of 1801, Part 1', *History Today*, 12 (February 1962), pp. 16–123.

—, 'The Egyptian Campaign of 1801, Part 2', *History Today*, (March 1962), pp. 177–86.

Chaplin, A., *Medicine in England during the Reign of George the Third* (London: published by the author, 1919).

Charles, C., 'Fergusson, William (1773–1846)', rev. J. Reznick, *ODNB*, online at http://www.oxforddnb.com/view/article/9339 [accessed 23 January 2008].

Charters, E. M., 'Disease, War, and the Imperial State: The Health of the British Armed Forces during the Seven Years War, 1756–63' (D.Phil dissertation, University of Oxford, 2006).

Chichester, H., 'Calvert, Sir Harry, first baronet (*bap.* 1763, *d.* 1826)', rev. J. Sweetman, *ODNB*, online at http://www.oxforddnb.com/view/article/4422 [accessed 16 March 2008].

Coley, N., 'Home, Sir Everard, first baronet (1756–1832)', *ODNB*, online at http://www.oxforddnb.com/view/article/13639 [accessed 16 March 2008].

Colley, L., *Britons, Forging the Nation 1707–1837*, 3rd edn (London: Yale University Press, 2005)

Cook, H. J., 'Practical Medicine and the British Armed Forces after the "Glorious Revolution"', *Medical History*, 34 (1990), pp. 1–26.

Cole, J. R., *Napoleon's Egypt: Invading the Middle East* (New York and Basingstoke: Palgrave MacMillan, 2007).

Cooter, R., 'Anticontagionism and History's Medical Record', in P. Wright and A. Treacher (eds), *The Problem of Medical Knowledge* (Edinburgh, 1982), pp. 87–108.

Creighton, C., 'Hunter, John (1754–1809)', rev. L. Wilkinson, *ODNB*, online at http://www.oxforddnb.com/view/article/14221 [accessed 16 March 2008].

Crowe, K., 'The Walcheren Expedition and the New Army Medical Board: A Reconsideration', *English Historical Review*, 88 (1973), pp. 770–85.

Courtney, W., 'Adams, Sir William (1783–1827)', rev. J. Tiffany, *ODNB*, online at http://www.oxforddnb.com/view/article/23200 [accessed 18 April 2006].

Database which formed the basis of M. Ackroyd, L. Brockliss, L., et al, *Advancing with the Army, Medicine, the Professions, and Social Mobility in the British Isles, 1790–1850* (Oxford, 2006). Held by Laurence W. B. Brockliss, Madgalen College, Oxford, OX1 4AU.

Davidson, L., '"Identities Ascertained": British Ophthalmology in the First Half of the Nineteenth Century', *Social History of Medicine*, 9 (1996), pp. 313–33.

Dible, J. H., *Napoleon's Surgeon* (London: Heinemann Medical, 1970).

Esdaile, C. J., *The Peninsular War: A New History* (London: Penguin, 2003).

Eighteenth Century Official Parliamentary Publications Portal 1688–1834, University of Southampton, online at http://www.parl18c.soton.ac.uk/parl18c/digbib/home.

Feibel, R., 'What Happened at Walcheren: The Primary Medical Sources', *Bulletin of the History of Medicine*, 42 (1968), pp. 62–79.

Finer, S. E., 'The Transmission of Benthamite Ideas 1820–50', in G. Sutherland (ed.), *Studies in the Growth of Nineteenth-Century Government* (London: Routledge and Kegan Paul, 1972), pp. 11–32.

Fisher, R. B., *Edward Jenner, 1749–1823* (London: Andre Deutsch, 1991).

Fissell, M. E., *Patients, Power, and the Poor in Eighteenth-Century Bristol* (Cambridge: Cambridge University Press, 1991).

Fortescue, J. W., *A History of the British Army*, 13 vols (London: Macmillan, 1910–30).

Foucault, M., *The Birth of the Clinic: An Archaeology of Medical Perception*, trans. A. M. Sheridan Smith (London: Tavistock, 1973).

Gascoigne, J., *Science in the Service of Empire, Joseph Banks, the British State and the uses of Science in the Age of Revolutions* (Cambridge: Cambridge University Press, 1998).

Gates, D. P., *The Spanish Ulcer, A History of the Peninsular War* (London: Pimlico, 2002).

Geggus, D. P., 'Yellow Fever in the 1790s: The British Army in Occupied Saint Domingue', *Medical History*, 23 (1979), pp. 38–58.

—, *Slavery, War and Revolution: The British Occupation of Saint Domingue 1793–1798* (Oxford and New York: Oxford University Press, 1982), pp. 347–72.

Giao, M., 'British Surgeons in the Portuguese Army during the Peninsular war', *Journal of the Royal Army Medical Corps*, 62 (1934), pp. 298–303.

Glover, M., *Wellington's Army in the Peninsula 1808–1814* (London and Vancouver: David & Charles, 1977).

—, *The Peninsular War, 1807–1814, A Concise Military History* (London: Penguin, 2001).

Gorin, G., *History of Ophthalmology* (Delaware: Publish or Perish, 1982).

Gruber, J., 'Hunter, John (1728–1793)', in H. Matthew and B. Harrison (eds), *ODNB*.

Hamlin, C., *Public Health and Social Justice in the Age of Chadwick, Britain, 1800–1854* (Cambridge: Cambridge University Press, 1998).

Harley, D., 'Rhetoric and the Social Construction of Sickness and Healing', *Social History of Medicine*, 12 (1999), pp. 407–35.

Harrison, M., 'Medicine and the Management of Modern Warfare', *History of Science*, 34 (1996), pp. 379–410.

—, *Climates and Constitutions: Health, Race, Environment and British Imperialism in India 1600–1850* (New Delhi: Oxford University Press, 1999).

—, 'Disease and Medicine in the Armies of British India, 1750–1830: The Treatment of Fevers and the Emergence of Tropical Therapeutics', in G. Hudson (ed.), *British Military and Naval Medicine, 1600–1830* (Amsterdam and New York: Rodopi, 2007), pp. 87–119.

—, 'From Medical Astrology to Medical Astronomy: Sol-Lunar and Planetary Theories of Disease in British Medicine, c. 1700–1850', *British Journal for the History of Science*, 33 (2000), pp. 25–48.

—, *Disease and the Modern World, 1500 to the Present Day* (Cambridge: Polity, 2004).

—, 'Maclean, Charles (fl. 1788–1824)', *ODNB*, online at http://www.oxforddnb.com/view/article/17649 [accessed 24 May 2006].

—, *Medicine in the Age of Commerce and Empire: Britain and its Tropical Colonies 1660–1830* (Oxford: Oxford University Press, 2010).

Heaman, E. A., 'The Rise and Fall of Anticontagionism in France', *Canadian Bulletin of Medical History*, 12 (1995), pp. 3–25.

Hibbert, C., *Corunna* (Moreton-In-Marsh: Windrush, 1996).

Hirschberg, J., *The History of Ophthalmology Translated by Frederick C. Blodi, M. D.* (Bonn: Wayenborgh, 1985).

Howard, M. R., 'Medical Aspects of Sir John Moore's Corunna Campaign, 1808–1809', *Journal of the Royal Society of Medicine*, 84 (1991), pp. 299–302.

—, 'Walcheren 1809: A Medical Catastrophe', *British Medical Journal*, 319 (1999), pp. 1642–1645.

—, *Wellington's Doctors: The British Army Medical Services in the Napoleonic Wars* (Staplehurst: Spellmount, 2002).

Howell, W., 'Augustus Bozzi Granville – Journeyman Physician', *Canadian Medical Association Journal*, 25 (1931), pp. 719–25.

Hudson, G. L., 'Introduction, British Military and Naval Medicine, 1600–1830', in G. L. Hudson (ed.), *British Military and Naval Medicine, 1600–1830* (Amsterdam and New York: Rodopi, 2007), pp. 7–22.

Jabartî, A., *Napoleon in Egypt: Al-Jabartî's Chronicle of the French Occupation, 1798*, trans. Shmuel Moreh (Princeton, NJ, and New York: M. Wiener, 1995).

Jacyna, L. S., *Philosophic Whigs: Medicine, Science and Citizenship in Edinburgh, 1789–1848* (London: Routledge, 1994).

Jewson, N., 'Medical Knowledge and the Patronage System in Eighteenth Century England', *Sociology*, 8 (1974), pp. 369–85.

—, 'The Landed Elite and Political Authority in Britain ca. 1760–1850', *Journal of British Studies*, 29 (1990), pp. 53–79.

Kaufman, M. H, *Surgeons at War – Medical Arrangements for the Treatment of the Sick and Wounded in the British Army during the Late Eighteenth and Nineteenth Centuries* (Westport, CT: Greenwood Press, 2001).

—, *The Regius Chair of Military Surgery in the University of Edinburgh, 1806–55* (Amsterdam: Rodopi, 2003).

Kelly, C., '"Not from the College, but through the Public and the Legislature": Charles Maclean and the Relocation of Medical Debate in the Early 19th Century', *Bulletin of the History of Medicine*, 82 (2008), pp. 545–69.

Kelly, J., 'Fitzpatrick, Sir Jeremiah (*c.* 1740–1810)', in *ODNB*, online at http://www.oxforddnb.com/view/article/61603 [accessed 16 March 2008]

Kempthorne, G., 'The Medical Department of Wellington's Army, 1809–1814', *Journal of the Royal Army Medical Corps*, 54 (1930), pp. 65–72, 131–46, 212–19.

—, 'The Egyptian Campaign of 1801', *Journal of the Royal Army Medical Corps*, 55 (1930), pp. 217–30.

—, 'The Army Medical Services 1816–1825', *Journal of the Royal Army Medical Corps*, 60 (1933), pp. 299–310.

—, 'The Army Medical Services at Home and Abroad 1803-1808', *Journal of the Royal Army Medical Corps*, 61 (1933), pp. 144–50, 223–32.

—, 'The Walcheren Expedition and the Reform of the Medical Board, 1809', *Journal of the Royal Army Medical Corps*, 62 (1934), pp. 133–8.

Kiple, K. F., 'Race, War and Tropical Medicine in the Eighteenth-Century Caribbean', in D. Arnold (ed.), *Warm Climates and Western Medicine* (Amsterdam and Atlanta: Rodopi, 1996), pp. 65–79.

Kondratas, R., 'The Brunonian Influence on the Medical Thought and Practice of Joseph Frank', in W. F. Bynum and R. Porter (eds), *Brunonianism in Britain and Europe* (London: Wellcome Institute for the History of Medicine, 1988), pp. 75–88.

Lawrence, C., *Medicine and the Making of Modern Britain 1700–1920* (London: Routledge, 1994).

—, 'Disciplining Diseases: Scurvy, the Navy and Imperial Expansion, 1750–1825', in D. Miller and P. Reill (eds), *Visions of Empire* (Cambridge: Cambridge University Press, 1996), pp. 80–106.

Lawrence, S. C., *Charitable Knowledge: Hospital Pupils and Practitioners in Eighteenth-Century London* (Cambridge: Cambridge University Press, 1996).

Lloyd, C., and J. Coulter, *Medicine and the Navy, 1200-1900, 1714–1815*, 3 vols (Edinburgh: Livingstone, 1961), vol. 3.

Loudon, I., *Medical Care and the General Practitioner, 1750–1850* (Oxford: Clarendon Press, 1986).

MacDonagh, O., *The Inspector General: Sir Jeremiah Fitzpatrick and the Politics of Social Reform, 1783–1802* (London: Croom Helm, 1981).

McGuffie, T., 'The Walcheren Expedition and the Walcheren Fever', *English Historical Review*, 62 (1947), pp. 191–202.

Macksey, P., *British Victory in Egypt, 1801: The End of Napoleon's Conquest* (London: Routledge, 1995).

Mathias, P., 'Swords into Ploughshares: The Armed Forces, Medicine and Public Health in the Late Eighteenth Century', in J. Winter (ed.), *War and Economic Development: Essays in Memory of David Joslin* (Cambridge: Cambridge University Press, 1975), pp. 73–90.

Meyerhof, M., 'A Short History of Ophthalmia during the Egyptian Campaigns of 1798–1807', *British Journal of Ophthalmology*, 16 (1932), pp. 138–47.

Moore, N., 'Pepys, Sir Lucas, first baronet (1742–1830)', rev. K. Bagshaw, *ODNB*, online at http://www.oxforddnb.com/view/article/21904 [accessed 14 March 2008].

Niebyl, P., 'The English Bloodletting Revolution, or Modern Medicine before 1850', *Bulletin of the History of Medicine*, 51 (1977), pp. 464–83.

Oman, C. W. C., *A History of the Peninsular War* (Oxford: Clarendon Press, 1902–30).

Oxford Dictionary of National Biography, available online at http://www.oxforddnb.com.

Pelling, M., 'Compromised by Gender: The Role of the Male Medical Practitioners in Early Modern England', in H. Marland and M. Pelling (eds), *The Task of Healing, Medicine, Religion and Gender in England and the Netherlands, 1450–1800* (Rotterdam: Erasmus, 1996), pp. 101–33.

Peterkin, A., W. Johnston and R. Drew, *Commissioned Officers in the Medical Services of the British Army, 1660–1960* (London: Wellcome Historical Medical Library, 1968).

Pickstone, J. V., 'Dearth, Dirt and Fever Epidemics: Rewriting the History of British "Public Health", 1780-1850', in T. Ranger and P. Slack (eds), *Epidemics and Ideas, Essays on the Historical Perception of Pestilence* (Cambridge: Cambridge University Press, 1992), pp. 125–48.

Richardson, R. G., *Larrey, Surgeon to Napoleon's Imperial Guard* (London: Quiller Press, 2000).

Rosen, G., *The Specialization of Medicine with Particular Reference to Ophthalmology* (New York: Froben Press, 1944).

Rosner, L., *Medical Education in the Age of Improvement: Edinburgh Students and Apprentices, 1760–1826* (Edinburgh: Edinburgh University Press, 1991).

—, *The Most Beautiful Man in Existence: The Scandalous Life of Alexander Lesassier* (Philadelphia: University of Pennsylvania Press, 1999).

Saakwa-Mante, N., 'Jackson, Robert (*bap.* 1750, *d.* 1827)', *ODNB*, online at http://www.oxforddnb.com/view/article/14547 [accessed 16 March 2008].

Sainty, J., *The Origin of the Office of Chairman of Committees in the House of Lords* (House of Lords Record Office, 1974), online at http://www.Parliament.uk/documents/upload/chairmn.pdf [accessed 7 July 2007].

Shapin, S., *A Social History of Truth: Civility and Science in Seventeenth-Century England* (Chicago, IL: University of Chicago Press, 1994).

Simms, B., 'Britain & Napoleon', *Historical Journal*, 41 (1998), pp. 885–94.

Stronach, G., 'Smyth, James Carmichael (1742–1821)', rev. J. Loudon, *ODNB*, online at http://www.oxforddnb.com/view/article/25950 [accessed 8 April 2008].

Thorne, R. G. (ed.), *The History of Parliament: House of Commons 1790–1820* (London: Secker & Warburg for the History of Parliament Trust, 1986).

Times Digital Archive, 1785–1985, Thompson Gale Databases.

Tröhler, U., *'To Improve the Evidence of Medicine': The 18th Century British Origins of a Critical Approach* (Edinburgh: Royal College of Physicians of Edinburgh, 2000).

United Kingdom Parliament website, online at http://www.parliament.uk/.

Vess, D., *Medical Revolution in France, 1789–1796* (Gainsville, FL: University Presses of Florida, 1975).

Wagemans M., and O. van Bijsterveld, 'The French Egyptian Campaign and its Effects on Ophthalmology', *Documenta Ophthalmologica*, 68 (1988), pp. 135–44.

Wallace, J., 'Blane, Sir Gilbert, first baronet (1749–1834)', *ODNB*, online at http://www. oxforddnb.com/view/article/2621 [accessed 30 September 2008].

Ward, S. G. P., *Wellington's Headquarters: A Study of the Administrative Problems in the Peninsula, 1809–1814* (London: Oxford University Press, 1957).

Watts, J., 'George James Guthrie, Peninsular Surgeon', *Proceedings of the Royal Society of Medicine* (1961), pp. 764–8.

Weisz, G., 'The Emergence of Specialization in the Nineteenth Century', *Bulletin of the History of Medicine*, 77 (2003), pp. 536–75.

Wellington Papers Database, University of Southampton, online at http://www.archives. soton.ac.uk/wellington/.

INDEX